Contemporary Topics
in Immunobiology
Volume 1

CONTEMPORARY TOPICS IN IMMUNOBIOLOGY

Contemporary Topics in Immunobiology

Volume 1

Edited by M. G. Hanna, Jr.

Oak Ridge National Laboratory
Oak Ridge, Tennessee

PLENUM PRESS • NEW YORK – LONDON • 1972

First Printing – January 1972
Second Printing – January 1974

Library of Congress Catalog Card Number 68-26769
ISBN 0-306-37801-9

© 1972 Plenum Press, New York
A Division of Plenum Publishing Corporation
227 West 17th Street, New York, N.Y. 10011

United Kingdom edition published by Plenum Press, London
A Division of Plenum Publishing Company, Ltd.
Davis House (4th Floor), 8 Scrubs Lane, Harlesden, NW10 6SE,
London, England

Printed in the United States of America

Contributors to This Volume

R. L. Carter *Chester Beatty Research Institute, Institute of Cancer Research: Royal Cancer Hospital, London, England*

Jacques M. Chiller *Department of Experimental Pathology, Scripps Clinic and Research Foundation, La Jolla, California*

Max D. Cooper *Spain Research Laboratories, Departments of Pediatrics and Microbiology, University of Alabama Medical Center, Birmingham, Alabama*

A. J. S. Davies *Chester Beatty Research Institute, Institute of Cancer Research: Royal Cancer Hospital, London, England*

Paul W. Kincade *Spain Research Laboratories, Departments of Pediatrics and Microbiology, University of Alabama Medical Center, Birmingham, Alabama*

Alexander R. Lawton *Spain Research Laboratories, Departments of Pediatrics and Microbiology, University of Alabama Medical Center, Birmingham, Alabama*

Victor Nussenzweig *Department of Pathology, New York University School of Medicine, New York, New York*

Carolyn S. Pincus *Department of Pathology, New York University School of Medicine, New York, New York*

George W. Santos *Division of Oncology, Department of Medicine, The Johns Hopkins University and Oncology Service, Baltimore City Hospitals, Baltimore, Maryland*

Noel L. Warner *Laboratory of Immunogenetics, The Walter and Eliza Hall Institute of Medical Research, Melbourne, Australia*

William O. Weigle *Department of Experimental Pathology, Scripps Clinic and Research Foundation, La Jolla, California*

Preface

Investigators, teachers, and practitioners in the biomedical sciences are keenly aware of the current crisis in scientific communications. With well over a thousand biomedical journals producing new issues each month, and with approximately five hundred new technical books in biomedicine being published each year,[1] not to mention the proliferation of information-exchange meetings, it is all too clear that we are in danger of being inundated by a flood of tables, figures, and hypotheses. The problem is particularly acute in immunology, as the rate of information production is increasing geometrically, and immunological approaches have been extended into other biological and medical fields to further diversify the research over a vast literature. Abstracting and information-retrieval services do much to improve the investigator's lot, but do not offer solutions for one particularly distressing aspect of the crisis. In the midst of our informational overabundance, one often finds that interrelationships between an investigator's collective findings are becoming blurred, or that the relation of his total work to the field are not clear. Although review articles are indispensable in fixing the status of a given problem, they do not provide the detailed attention to a single author's work that is needed.

A consensus of the editors associated with this new publication series in immunology was that what is lacking in the literature is an outlet that allows a single investigator or research group to develop in one chapter a summary of individual works published over a period of years and distributed in various journals. Such an outlet would be especially important if the authors have achieved a "critical mass" of data and have completed, over several years of study, definitive experiments that consolidate a new working hypothesis or that modify or disprove an existing working hypothesis. It is anticipated that such articles would be presented in a concise manner, unburdened by tangential issues. In this way authors could reevaluate important aspects of their studies in the light of pertinent recent literature, and provide a perspective of

---

[1]Orr, R. H., and Leeds, A., 1964. Biomedical literature: Volume, growth and other characteristics. *Federation Proceedings*, **23**:1310-1331.

the usefulness of their ideas in applied immunology. Such is the goal of *Contemporary Topics in Immunobiology*.

It is anticipated that each year pairs of editors will work together to develop a volume that will reflect their areas of interest and expertise. The selection of authors will be made by the two editors, relying on their individual and joint knowledge of advances in the field of immunology.

The first volume is two things. It is, first, a "syntopicon" that provides the spectrum of interest of the associate editors of the series, and, second, an indication of the style and format of the entire series. In Chapter 1, "Systems of Lymphocytes in Mouse and Man: An Interim Appraisal," Davies and Carter have done a remarkable job of evaluating contemporary cellular immunology. Besides relating essential experimental findings on B- and T-cell systems of lymphocytes in terms of organization, interaction, and function, they have attempted to establish a greater relevance, to clinical medicine, of the results from the experimental systems. While they point out that the evidence for B- and T-cell systems in man is almost entirely inferential at the present time, they attempt to relate the known functional activities of this system to congenital immune deficiency state and lymphoid neoplasia in man. The presentation stresses that greater knowledge of these lymphoid systems has a tremendous potential advantage to clinical medicine and encourages immunologists to be conscious of the need to establish a wider relevance of results obtained from experimental systems.

In Chapter 2, "A Developmental Approach to the Biological Basis for Antibody Diversity," Cooper, Lawton, and Kincaid present new insights into the origin, identity, and characteristics of pre-antibody-forming cells. The important results presented in this paper argue that the developmental basis of antibody diversity is associated with the interrelationship between the immunocompetent progenitor cells or stem cells and the microenvironment in which the cell differentiation is initiated. The authors state, further, that immunoglobulin synthesis appears to be "a normal event in cellular differentiation rather than one that is dependent on the influence of exogenous antigens," and that the early synthesis of immunoglobulin fulfills the role of cell membrane "recognition antibodies." The data relevant to this interpretation is obtained in the chicken, a favorite experimental system because the site of induction of stem cells along antibody-producing lines is in the bursa of Fabricius, an accessible and central lymphoepithelial organ. A question still may be raised as to whether this model, developed from the bursa of Fabricius in the chicken, has relevance to plasma cell differentiation in mammals—which brings up the classic controversy concerning the mammalian bursa equivalent, a topic dealt with in depth by Cooper and Lawton in Chapter 3, "The Mammalian 'Bursa Equivalent': Does Lymphoid Differentiation along Plasma Cell Lines Begin in the Gut-Associated Lymphoepithelial Tissues (GALT) of Mammals?"

In Chapter 4, "C3-Receptor Sites on Leukocytes: Possible Role in Opsonization and the Immune Response," Nussenzweig and Pincus assemble the results of several years of work in their laboratory to provide new insight into specific recognition units on lymphocyte plasma membranes. They demonstrate how these markers on lymphocytes permit the separation of cells into subpopulations which probably have distinct functions in the immune response. Specifically, the properties of receptors for immunoglobulin and complement components on the membrane of lymphocytes are evaluated as to specific recognition by lymphocytes of antigen-antibody interaction leading to complement fixation. They discuss how the demonstrated receptors for modified C3 on the membrane of lymphocytes relate to basic mechanisms of the immune response as well as lymphocyte proliferation.

The fact that receptor sites, acting as recognition units on lymphocyte plasma membranes, is a contemporary area of research for immunologists as well as cell biologists is emphasized in Chapter 5. Noel Warner's discussion of surface immunoglobulins on lymphoid cells concentrates on two key questions: (1) Is the immunoglobulin detected on surface of B-lymphocytes the actual antigen-binding receptors? (2) Do immunoglobulin receptors exist on T-lymphocytes, and if so, are they antigen receptors? The discussion of these questions is based on Warner's current approaches to this problem. Of extreme interest in this chapter is Warner's integration of the current work of antigen-binding lymphocytes and antigen "suicidal" killing of lymphocytes with the functional and physiologic processes associated with immunoglobulin surface receptors. He also attempts to incorporate the available data into a working hypothesis regarding immunoglobulin expression in lymphoid cell differentiation, which raised several questions as well as approaches to elaborate the actual nature and number of immunoglobulin classes that are expressed by B- and T-cells during differentiation, and regarding what effect antigen stimulation has on the type and amount of immunoglobulins synthesized.

Chapter 6 by Chiller and Weigle discusses one of the most critical questions existing today in immunology, the question of the cellular basis of immunological unresponsiveness. The chapter emphasizes the cellular phenomena involved in the induction, maintenance, and termination of immunological unresponsiveness as it specifically relates to the block in the formation of humoral antibody. Besides a remarkable integration of their extensive data with data from other laboratories, these authors carefully discuss the techniques of preparation and characteristics of various immunogens and tolerogens, as well as their use in various immune systems. Their data strongly suggest that "tolerant animals may possess the full potential to produce antibody specific to the tolerated antigen, but fail to recognize the antigen as an immunogenic molecule." On the basis of current understanding of cell collaboration in the immune system, they are tempted to view the cellular dynamics involved in unresponsiveness as selective unresponsiveness of T-cells without concomitant tolerance in B-cells.

In Chapter 7, "Applications of Marrow Grafts in Human Disease: Its Problems and Potential," Santos provides a personal appraisal derived from 15 years of laboratory and clinical studies of bone marrow transplantation. His discussion outlines the rationale, potential, and some of the problems associated with application of marrow grafts in human disease. Also, a benefit derived from this discussion is the extensive experimental and clinical experience with chemically induced immune suppression, as well as the nature and control of graft-versus-host disease. The development and complexities of the lymphohematopoietic system as they relate to marrow transplantation is also presented. Marrow transplantation as a prelude to organ grafts and as a treatment in malignancy is also outlined. It is in an area such as this that the impact of the wider relevance of immunology will be experienced.

I wish to thank the associate editors for their cooperation and to express optimism and great anticipation for the future volumes of this series. Tentatively, it is considered that Volume 2 will be organized by A. J. S. Davies and R. L. Carter, and Volume 3 by M. D. Cooper and N. L. Warner.

M. G. Hanna, Jr.
General Editor

Contents

Chapter 1

Systems of Lymphocytes in Mouse and Man: An Interim Appraisal

A. J. S. Davies and R. L. Carter
Chester Beatty Research Institute
Institute of Cancer Research: Royal Cancer Hospital
London, England

INTRODUCTION

Advances in immunology are taking place with an increasing tempo and on a broadening front. Progress has been particularly marked in the field of cellular immunology, where much effort is being directed toward identifying the origins of cells which take part in immune responses. The different contributions made by immunologists, developmental biologists, geneticists, biochemists, and pathologists are disclosing a situation of considerable complexity, and the occasional reviewer cannot hope to produce more than an interim account. In the present review, we shall concentrate mainly on current theories that deal with the origin, structure, and functional organization of the mammalian system of lymphocytes. Although the emphasis will be on the experimental animal rather than man, we are very conscious of the need to establish the wider relevance of results obtained from such experimental systems. We believe that these results are not (in W. H. Auden's phrase) "abstract models of events, derived from dead experiments," and we shall consider some of their clinical implications in the last section of this review.

CHOICE OF WORKING MATERIALS

It is commonly held that the contributions made by the experimental immunologist and the clinical immunologist are (or should be) complementary and that a combined approach is potentially the most fruitful way to attack many immunological problems. It is doubtful whether fundamental differences exist between biological systems in man and in other animals, and the use of mammalian models with which to examine detailed aspects of the lymphocyte system seems a legitimate course of action. Experimental cellular immunology relies heavily on work with small rodents, particularly inbred and coisogenic strains of mice in which the histocompatibility genes are well characterized. Chromosomally marked strains of mice are available, and the genetic determination of the immunoglobulin allotypes is fairly well understood in some species, particularly in rabbits.

IN VITRO SYSTEMS

Various in vitro systems are available, the principal ones deriving either from the spleen suspension culture methods of Mishell and Dutton (1967) or from the organ culture methods of Globerson and Auerbach (1966). In addition, it has become common practice to culture peripheral blood lymphocytes in vitro, often in the presence of mitogenic agents (Nowell, 1960) such as phytohemagglutinin (PHA). A number of methods have been devised by which immune functions of individual cells and cell populations can be estimated in vitro, for example, the Jerne plaque technique (Jerne and Nordin, 1963), and the various rosette-forming cell determinations (Zaalberg, 1964; Bach et al., 1970).

Sophisticated in vitro methods have been developed to separate lymphoid cells on the basis of characteristics such as cell surface charges (Hannig and Zeiller, 1969), buoyant density (Raidt et al., 1968), and specific adherence to antigen (Wigzell and Andersson, 1969). Apart from these techniques of separation, other methods have emerged for identification on the basis of cell surface antigens (Reif and Allen, 1964; Raff, 1969) (see below). But despite the variety of techniques available, it has not always proved easy to ascertain what in vivo phenomena are reflected in the behavior of lymphoid cells growing in tissue culture vessels.

IN VIVO METHODS

Several groups of investigators have concentrated on experiments with more or less intact animals, often using irradiated animals as recipients of lymphoid cells, the functional potentiality of which can subsequently be tested in various ways (Harris et al., 1954; Davies et al., 1967). A number of methods have been used to identify the transferred cells, including antigenic

(Gengozian *et al.*, 1957), biochemical (van Bekkum and Vos, 1957), and chromosomal markers (Ford *et al.*, 1956).

Burnet (1970) has described many of these relatively new methods as "extremely elaborate and artificial," but they have unquestionably aided our understanding of the lymphoid system and its function.

Other workers, notably Good and his associates, have concentrated on the various immunological deficiency syndromes encountered in clinical medicine—the so-called experiments of nature (e.g., Peterson *et al.*, 1965). Much useful information has emerged, some of which is discussed later on p. 18; but for the moment we are concerned principally with analyzing the lymphoid system in the experimental animal rather than man.

PRIMARY AND SECONDARY LYMPHOID ORGANS

In developmental terms, the lymphoid organs of mammals can be regarded as primary or secondary (Miller and Davies, 1964). The thymus and the bursa of Fabricius (in birds) are described as primary lymphoid organs; the spleen and lymph nodes comprise secondary lymphoid organs. In addition to their developmental connotation, the terms *primary* and *secondary* imply that the growth and activities of the primary lymphoid organs precede the full development and maturation of secondary lymphoid structures. More specifically, there is increasing evidence that cells derived from the thymus and bursa seed the secondary lymphoid organs, where they play a role in immunological responses. It is suspected on indirect evidence (e.g., Glick *et al.*, 1956) that bursal cells have the capacity to develop into plasma cells and synthesize humoral antibody in response to appropriate antigenic stimuli, whereas thymus-derived lymphoid cells are concerned with cell-mediated immune responses of the delayed hypersensitivity type. This apparently clear dichotomy of thymus and bursa, each organ supplying functionally distinct cells to the secondary lymphoid organs, is compatible with many observations from the clinical immune deficiency syndromes, and it is pleasingly symmetrical; but it is unsatisfactory for a number of reasons. It takes no account of the sources of cells going to the primary lymphoid organs. Also, it is by no means clear whether there is a discrete bursal equivalent in the mammal.

Despite obvious deficiencies in our knowledge, there has been a tendency to establish a definitive picture of the lymphoid system. This tendency is in keeping with the tradition of basing progress on a working hypothesis, but we need to remember that disproof of any working hypothesis is as important as its consolidation. From various experimental systems, however, some facts are emerging which can be used to build up at least a provisional and impressionist picture of both the development and maintenance of the lymphoid system.

DEVELOPMENT OF THE LYMPHOID SYSTEM:
PRECURSOR CELL MIGRATIONS

In mice, it appears that progenitor cells (probably arising in the vicinity of the primitive streak) recirculate in the early stages of embryonic life. Some of these lodge in the thymus, where they proliferate and probably differentiate as well (Moore and Owen, 1967). The progeny, an unknown number of cell generations away from their precursor, leave the thymus and enter the circulation. In the mouse this process of seeding from the thymus probably starts at about the eighteenth day of gestation (Owen and Ritter, 1969). Since the first precursor cells enter the thymus at about the eleventh day (Moore and Owen, 1967), it appears that thymus processing can take as little as 7 days. It is, however, uncertain whether 7 days is an average value, and it cannot be assumed that the first cells to leave the thymus are necessarily descended from the first precursor cells to enter the organ. Nor is it known whether the pace of thymus processing varies according to the physiological condition of the animal. It is broadly assumed that precursor cells continue to enter the thymus as the organism matures, but proof of this proposition relies heavily at present on experiments with irradiated animals which may well create artifacts that are not necessarily relevant to the normal condition. "Normality" in relation to the lymphoid tissue is depressingly difficult to define and even more difficult to experiment upon without creating more or less unnatural disturbances.

It is no part of current dogma that lymphocytes arise by proliferative activity of the thymic epithelial cells. It is assumed that the thymus processing involves division of the precursor cells, partly because mitotic figures are common in the thymus and partly because grafted thymuses can still grow from small numbers of residual cells (Leuchars et al., 1967). Other evidence shows that cells which have synthesized DNA in the thymus, and which are therefore supposedly part of a mitotic compartment, do leave the organ (Nossal and Gorrie, 1964). It must, however, be admitted that cells could enter the thymus and undergo differentiation without mitosis; none of the methods of investigation presently available precludes this possibility.

It is part of the current theory that the precursor cells enter the thymus (through an unknown portal) and that processing begins in the outer regions of the cortex. With time and intervening mitosis, the progeny cells pass to the deeper parts of the cortex, finally coming to rest as "mature" cells in the medulla (Borum, 1968; Köbberling, 1965; Hinrichsen, 1965; Slonecker et al., 1969). They probably leave the medulla either in the venous sinuses (as in the spleen) or in efferent lymphatics (as in lymph nodes), or by both routes. Metcalf (1966) has postulated that many of the cells generated in the thymus normally die there, but there is little histological evidence for such a graveyard phenomenon. Others have suggested that only 20-30% of the cells produced in the thymus leave it in the venous blood (Ernström and Sandberg, 1970). This is a difficult field of investigation, and, despite early precedents (Hewson, 1777) for supposing that lymphocytes leave the thymus in large numbers, it is doubtful that we shall discover their exact route(s) of exit for some time.

SURFACE ANTIGEN CHANGES

Certain changes in antigens at the cell surface have been detected during thymus processing (Lance et al., 1971; Raff, 1971; Owen and Raff, 1970). The lymphoid precursor cell itself is thought to lack the θ antigen, but it develops a high degree of θ positivity fairly soon after entering the thymus. This acquisition of θ antigen is, however, apparently short-lived, and much of the antigen seems to be lost toward the end of differentiation. These changes have been described in experiments in which suspensions of thymic cells have been mixed with cytotoxic antisera, and it would be of interest to use the same sera in combination with fluorescent antiglobulin antisera on intact thymic tissue in histological sections. Broadly comparable changes have been found with the TL antigen, which can be demonstrated on about 90% of thymic lymphocytes in certain strains of mice. As lymphocytes external to the thymus are normally TL-negative in these animals, it seems likely that the loss of TL positivity in the thymus is associated with maturation. The significance of such changes in surface antigenicity is not known.

EXTRATHYMIC MATURATION

Argument continues over whether the cells which leave the thymus are already mature or whether they undergo some extrathymic maturation. Many experiments have been performed in which the functional capacities of thymocytes (usually in immune responses) have been tested, but little attention has been paid to the state of differentiation of these prematurely released cells; most investigators have simply equated them with T cells external to the thymus.

In addition to the problem of processing within the thymus, there is the question of the fate of cells which are normally released from the thymus and enter the T-cell pool. It has been argued that relatively few of these survive for long (Davies et al., 1971), and at present there is much argument about factors which might promote T-cell survival. The most likely of these is contact with antigen, but a post-thymic humoral influence from the thymus is an additional possibility.

T-CELL POOL AND RECIRCULATION

T cells external to the thymus probably form the bulk of a recirculating pool of lymphocytes, the existence of which was first established by Gowans (1959). Once the T cell has left the thymus and is fully mature, it is a cell with a relatively long intermitotic interval which, at any moment in time, will be either in the bloodstream or in the lymphoid tissues (particularly in the interfollicular cortex of nodes or the periarteriolar regions of the spleen). T cells probably leave the bloodstream through the postcapillary venules in lymph nodes and return to it in the efferent lymphatics. It is not known whether there is an equivalent of the postcapillary venule in the spleen, but it seems likely that lymphocytes emerge into the marginal sinuses and from there move inward towards the central arteriole. Their subsequent fate has not been determined, but it is commonly assumed that some mechanism operates by which the cells are carried out into the venous collecting sinuses of the red pulp; there may be a special point of exit of such cells from the lymphoid follicles.

The nature of the interaction between the T cell and the endothelial cells of the postcapillary venules (or their splenic equivalents) is uncertain, although it appears that the lymphocyte can either penetrate the capillary wall (Marchesi and Gowans, 1964) or migrate through the intercellular junctions (Morris, 1968) in a manner broadly similar to that of granulocytes leaving the circulation at points of inflammation (Florey, 1970).

There is information which suggests that antigenic stimuli can alter the rate of emergence of cells from the bloodstream into a draining lymph node (Morris, 1968). Studies of the flow of efferent lymph from a lymph node have, however, demonstrated various alterations in cellular output when the node is stimulated antigenically (Hall and Morris, 1965), and similar observations have been made with spleens maintained *in vitro* on a cell circulation pump into which antigen has been introduced (Ford, 1969).

Little is known of the entry of T cells into the nonlymphoid tissues and their subsequent drainage into lymph nodes via afferent lymphatics, but it should be stressed that extravascular lymphocytes are common in tissues and that such cells constitute an important part of the total lymphocyte pool.

ORGAN DISTRIBUTION OF T CELLS

Analysis of the distribution of T cells by studying the density of θ-positive cells indicates that there are rather fewer T cells in polysynthetic nodes (Raff and Wortis, 1970), which are broadly those associated with drainage of the alimentary canal, than in oligosynthetic nodes, which characteristically

drain regions where there is not continuous antigenic stimulation. This observation tallies with the suggestion that T cells are not mitotically active con-
stituents of the germinal centers which are a common feature of polysynthetic
nodes (Koller et al., 1966). However, it may be that the polysynthetic lymph
nodes act as a bursal equivalent—we shall return to this point. A disturbing
alternative possibility is that T-cell surface antigenicity is not expressed to the
same degree in T cells which are responding to antigenic stimulation.

   The exact role of T cells in the immune response is still a question for
argument. It has been demonstrated that T cells in regional lymph nodes
respond by mitosis to a variety of antigenic stimuli which include sheep red
blood cells (Davies et al., 1969b), oxazolone (Davies et al., 1969a), and skin
homografts (Davies et al., 1966). When this mitotic response is sufficiently
large, it is accompanied by hyperplasia of the paracortical zone in the associated nodes (Davies et al., 1969a). It thus seems that T cells in the thymus-
dependent areas (Parrott et al., 1966) respond to the presence of antigen by
undergoing mitosis, but this conclusion must be adopted with some caution as
the correlation between histological appearance and the cytological analysis
required to define T-cell mitotic activity (see below) is only approximate.

   It is not known where in the lymphoid system (or outside it) antigen
and T cells meet, and the significance of T-cell mitosis following antigenic
stimulation is also obscure. It could be that more T cells capable of perform-
ing a specific function are produced—a simple amplification mechanism. Alternatively, the very considerable changes which occur in the surfaces and enzyme content of dividing T cells may be relevant to the expression of their
cooperative function. It has been shown in many experimental systems that T
cells cooperate with other lymphoid cells in the production of humoral antibody (Claman et al., 1966; Davies et al., 1967; Mitchell and Miller, 1968), but
neither the mechanism, nor the site, nor the biological significance of this
synergism has yet been established.

B CELLS

   So far we have only written of the development of T cells, but there is
fairly widespread agreement that at least one other developmental pathway
exists. In the adult mouse there is a second population of lymphoid cells
which is thought to be derived ultimately from the bone marrow, the so-called
B cells (Roitt et al., 1969). (This term is, however, ambiguous, as some writers
use B cells to indicate an origin from bursal elements.) It seems likely that
there are some circulating B-cell precursors in the blood because injection of
peripheral blood leukocytes into irradiated mice is an effective therapeutic
expedient—effective because hematopoietic function, including lymphocyte

production, accrues from the injected cells (C. E. Ford, personal communication). There was no specific demonstration of B cells in these experiments, but it is unlikely that an animal can survive without B Cells and it seems reasonable to assume that their precursors were present among the injected cell populations. It is, however, difficult at present to adduce information about the development of the B-cell population in the embryo. At the time that lymphocytes are first seen in the thymus there do not appear to be any other lymphocytes present in the body. Soon after birth in mice there is a rapid increase in the number of lymphocytes in peripheral lymphoid organs. This can be accounted for in part by an increase in the number of "processed" T cells discharged from the thymus, but it must also be assumed that considerable numbers of B cells are produced at the same time. Unlike T cells, B cells probably tend not to recirculate but remain in the outer follicular regions of lymph nodes and splenic follicles and in medullary cords. It is widely thought that, unlike T cells, B cells are a "short-lived" species. This view is almost certainly wrong in conditions of continuous or repeated antigenic stimulation, where there is evidence that specifically stimulated B cells may become a persistent population (Askonas et al., 1970; Askonas, personal communication). The one fairly certain characteristic of B cells is their capacity to produce and secrete antibody, which the present dogma does not accept as a property of the T cells.

Many provisos must, however, be made about this idealized concept of the B cell. Firstly, it is not known whether B-cell production and behavior are affected by the general presence of T cells. In the specific instance of cooperation, it is clear that the two cells interact, but it is not certain whether such interactions directly or indirectly affect B-cell turnover. Secondly, we do not know whether all B cells derive directly from the bone marrow or whether some B-cell precursors from the bone marrow proliferate and mature in peripheral lymphoid organs. Hall and Morris (1964) showed that locally irradiated nodes are quickly repopulated by circulating cells without any evidence of mitotic regeneration within the node; this finding does not preclude the possibility that under normal circumstances some lymphocytes are produced in the node itself.

In his classical studies on the lymphoid system, Yoffey distinguished between oligo- and polysynthetic lymph nodes (Yoffey and Olson, 1966). In the former, mitotic figures and germinal centers are rare; in the latter—usually associated with the alimentary canal—both germinal centers and mitotic figures are more common. As germinal centers are uncommon in germ-free mice and the development of the gut-associated lymphoid tissue is limited, it is reasonable to suppose that the existence of germinal centers and the number of lymphocytes present within them reflects a continuous immunological reaction to the various antigenic components of the contents of the gut. This conclusion is in keeping with the many demonstrations that germinal centers are commonly produced after antigenic stimulation.

Many attempts have been made to establish the function of germinal centers. They were originally described as sites for lymphocytopoiesis; more recently they were regarded as regions which become active during an immune response and where either antibody-forming cells and/or memory cells are produced (see Cottier et al., 1967). No definitive evidence for any of these notions has emerged, although it is known that both antigen and specific antibody can be readily localized within germinal centers by immunofluorescence and other techniques and that the germinal centers contain special dendritic macrophages which trap antigen (Ada et al., 1967; Hunter et al., 1969; Hanna et al., 1969).

It is convenient to suppose that in addition to the specific function of individual germinal centers, they are a uniform collection of organs for which an overall common function(s) can also be specified. We suggest for heuristic reasons that germinal centers are sites at which nonspecific amplification of the B-cell precursor populations can occur. The proliferation is induced by antigen-antibody complexes held in the germinal centers, and the gut-associated lymphoid tissues would have a special part to play in any such amplification because they normally contain the bulk of germinal centers. This suggestion owes much to discussion with Dr. B. H. Waksman, and the notion is implicit in one of his earlier considerations of the possible significance of lymphoid tissue in the appendix of the rabbit (Ozer and Waksman, 1970).

At this point a digression must be made briefly to consider the nature and significance of the bursa of Fabricius in the chicken. The bursa is an organized lymphoid organ which develops as an evagination from the rectum. Its removal drastically impairs the capacity of the bird to produce humoral antibody (Warner and Szenberg, 1964). It has been suggested that the bursa, like the thymus, is a differentiating environment in which lymphoid cells acquire certain specialized functions. In the case of cells which derive from the bursa, this function is the synthesis and release of antibody in response to an appropriate antigenic stimulus. It is not certain whether cooperation between T cells and bursal cells occurs at all in birds; indeed, extreme protagonists of the theory that bursa and thymus represent two different branches of the same developmental tree would claim that such cooperation is neither found nor necessary. There is some debate as to whether cells develop de novo within the bursa or whether this organ acts as a processing environment for cells derived from elsewhere; the latter is probably correct (Moore and Owen, 1967). Young birds differ from mammals in that they have no discrete lymph nodes, the only major accumulations of organized lymphoid tissue being the spleen, bursa, and thymus. Despite these uncertainties, there have been vigorous attempts to find a bursal equivalent in the mammal. The possibility of regulating the capacity to produce humoral antibody by manipulation of one discrete organ has considerable appeal. The tonsils, caecal appendix, and Peyer's patches have all been proposed for this role on more or less tenuous grounds, but there is no unanimity of opinion.

The present hypothesis concerning the amplification of B cells in germinal centers is an attempt to reconcile those who espouse the bursal equivalent theory (*B cell* was coined to indicate *b*ursal equivalent) and those who resolutely reject it as a concept of any usefulness in mammals. It is pleasing on the grounds of symmetry to suppose that the mature B and T lymphocytes in the mammal derive from common ancestral stem cells in the bone marrow. Such precursor cells would undergo amplification and differentiation in either the thymus or in germinal centers. The precursor cells could initially undergo either form of differentiation, but it is likely that their capacity to do so would be reduced with increasing numbers of cell generations—phenotypic flexibility is thus limited by generational age. The principal uncertainty about such a hypothesis is whether the stage at which the B cell or its precursor leaves the bone marrow is equivalent to that of the T cell when it leaves the thymus. Brahim and Osmond (1970) have presented evidence that cells with the morphology of small lymphocytes are produced in the bone marrow and then migrate to peripheral lymphoid organs. Such an observation is not incompatible with the present hypothesis, as the generational age of the emigrant cells has not been determined. If it were shown that the emigrant lymphocytes had very little capacity for further proliferation, the hypothesis would require modification.

A WORKING HYPOTHESIS

On the basis of the evidence presented so far, a working hypothesis can be formulated along the following lines: (1) The system of lymphocytes (at least in the adult mouse) consists of at least two distinguishable elements termed *T cells* and *B cells*. (2) B cells are a principal constituent of the cell populations in the outer follicular regions and medullary cords of lymph nodes, and in the splenic white pulp. (3) T cells are a principal constituent of the recirculating lymphocyte population and are particularly common in the periarteriolar sheaths of the splenic white pulp and in the interfollicular cortex of lymph nodes. (4) B cells are capable of the synthesis and secretion of antibody, but their capacity to do so is often augmented when they cooperate with T cells.

In order to use this working hypothesis to analyze the various ways in which the lymphoid system can be perturbed, it is necessary to have methods for quantitating B cells and T cells and their respective precursors, and also to have some indications of their turnover. It has been possible to devise ways of quantitating T cells and their precursors, but it is more difficult at the moment to apply similar methods to B cells. The methods discussed here represent attempts at quantitation of the T-cell population *en masse* based on common properties of the T cells and their precursors; this approach provides a structural rather than functional analysis of the lymphoid system.

METHODS OF QUANTITATION OF T CELLS

There are two principal ways to quantitate T cells at the present time: (1) on the basis of their surface antigens, and (2) in reconstitution experiments in which chromosomally distinguishable cell populations are used.

1. Reif and Allen (1964) described the θ antigen, which characterizes thymus and also brain cells in the mouse; recent evidence (Boyse *et al.*, 1970) suggests that skin epithelial cells may also be θ-positive. A small amount of the antigen was present in cells from peripheral lymphoid organs, but, although Reif and Allen thought that this material might be on cells of thymic origin external to the thymus, they did not have a suitable method for its quantitation. Raff (1969) and Raff and Wortis (1970) subsequently showed that Reif's suspicions were correct and that reasonably accurate quantitation of T cells could be achieved by measuring the release of isotopic chromium (Cr^{51}) from labeled lymphocytes treated with an anti-θ antisera. The θ antigen has been shown to have two isoantigenic variants, termed θ-C3H and θ-AKR. It is possible to construct radiation chimeras in which an adult mouse of either the C3H or AKR strain is thymectomized, irradiated, and reconstituted with syngeneic bone marrow and a neonatal thymus graft from the other strain. In such animals the thymus graft, after an early phase of partial involution, grows and releases cells which initially have the θ antigenicity of the thymus graft donor. Subsequently, the cells which emerge from the thymus carry the θ antigenicity of the bone-marrow donor. Theoretically, the replacement of the cohort of cells with the antigenicity of the thymus graft by cells from the bone marrow graft could provide a means of quantitation of T-cell pool maintenance. In addition, the rate of appearance of the cell population derived from bone marrow graft could be used as a measure of the T-cell precursors in the bone-marrow inoculum. With a knowledge of the distribution of θ antigens, it is thus possible to quantitate T-cell precursors, T-cell numbers, and T-cell pool maintenance. The most obvious objection is that the thymus graft in an allogeneic chimera might not function in a normal manner, but the C3H and AKR strains of mice have the same *H-2* genes (*H-2k*), and the evidence available indicates that such a difference does not lead to serious functional incompatibilities in chimeric situations.

2. The T6 chromosome marker was first discovered as a hemizygous reciprocal translocation in the progeny of some irradiated mice. It was established in the homozygous state in a random-bred strain of animals and was widely used as a means of tracing cells in the early studies of radiation chimeras. The Harwell group transferred the chromosome into the CBA/H strain of mice, and by a long series of backcrosses established an inbred CBA/H.*T6T6* substrain which is histocompatible with CBA/H but chromosomally distinguishable from it (Ford and Micklem, 1963). Numerous experiments have been made with these two strains, but our particular concern here is with studies in which CBA/H adult mice have been thymectomized, irradiated, and reconstituted with CBA/H bone marrow and a CBA/H.*T6T6* thymus graft. The development of the chimeric state in these animals is perhaps a partial re-enactment of the kind of developmental pathway by which the hematopoietic and lymphoid systems develop in the embryo. After a short phase of incomplete involution, the thymus graft grows vigorously for about 18 days by proliferation of the cells which were in the graft at the time of its transfer (Leuchars *et al.*, 1967). It is assumed that the residual cells are stem cells which had migrated into the thymus in its original host. After the eighteenth day, the population of dividing cells changes over within a few days so that cells from the bone marrow inoculum are thereafter the only cell type to be found (Leuchars *et al.*, 1967). (Very rarely mitotic figures are encountered which have the chromosomal phenotype of the native cell population; these are probably dividing epithelial cells as there is no evidence that the epithelial components of a thymus graft are replaced from outside.) From about the fifteenth day, cells with the graft marker can be found in the peripheral blood (Doenhoff and Davies, 1971), the chromosome markers being demonstrable *in vitro* in the presence of a mitogen such as phytohemagglutinin (PHA). These cells increase in number until about the 45th day, well beyond the time that the native cell populations can be found dividing in the graft itself (Doenhoff and Davies, 1971). Three conclusions may be drawn: either that considerable numbers of mature cells are retained in the graft for some time after the last mitosis which gave rise to them, or that a period of extrathymic maturation is necessary before cells can respond fully to PHA, or that there is some amplification of the T-cell population external to the thymus. On various counts this last alternative is unpopular, principally because adult thymectomized mice show a decline in immunological competence and peripheral blood lymphocyte levels (Jeejeebhoy, 1965; Metcalf, 1965; Miller, 1965; Taylor, 1965), and neonatally thymectomized animals rarely show any consistent spontaneous improvement in the condition of their lymphoid system. If T-cell populations expanded to fill the space available, following Parkinson's law, it might be supposed that adult thymectomized

mice would not show a decline in their lymphoid system nor would neonatally thymectomized animals remain immunologically incompetent. The possibility that T cells can maintain or expand their population size external to the thymus but only in the presence of the thymus cannot be excluded.

The proposal that cells are retained within the thymus has been established in a series of retransplantation experiments. Extrathymic maturation is at the moment an interesting theoretical possibility. The cohort of cells derived from the original cell population in the thymus graft can be followed for many months, and its replacement by cells of bone marrow origin is again a measure of T-cell pool maintenance.

T-cell precursors can be quantitated in a similar manner. When varying numbers of CBA/H.T6T6 bone marrow cells are injected into irradiated CBA/H mice (with their thymuses intact), the proportion of host:donor cells among a lymphocyte population examined 50 days after irradiation and cell transfer is linearly related (on a log plot) to the numbers of donor cells in the original inoculum (Doenhoff and Davies, 1971). The explanation of this finding is that cells derived from the injected bone marrow compete with the residual host cells in the thymus and that the eventual outcome of this competition is revealed in the composition of the T-cell population external to the thymus.

It can thus be seen that T cells, their precursors, and their turnover can all be monitored using either surface antigens or chromosome markers. The techniques involving chromosome markers are more laborious and are limited to cell populations which can be persuaded to enter mitosis. Methods involving surface antigens are technically more difficult and probably less accurate, but they give results more easily and quickly.

Raff et al., (1971) have shown that it is possible to identify mouse B cells by the use of a heterologous anti-MBLA (mouse-bone-marrow lymphocyte antigen) antiserum. This method should theoretically provide a ready means for quantitating B cells, but it has only recently been described and its general usefulness remains to be proved.

So far we have given a generalized account of the lymphoid system with a working hypothesis and described two methods for quantitation of the thymus-oriented part of the system. It now remains to outline an approach to further studies.

It is convenient to think of the lymphoid system as a discrete functional entity. It is also convenient to regard it as a system which is sensitive to various environmental factors and which has some capacity for autoregulation. Some of these environmental factors, such as the nutritional or hormonal state of the host organism, can be regarded as "internal"; others, outside the whole organism, can be thought of as "external."

AUTOREGULATION

Over the last few years an increasing number of humoral products of lymphoid cells have been discovered. Some of these materials, particularly antibodies, are specific to the inducing stimulus; others, such as interferon, are produced in response to a specific class of stimuli but lack the specificity of antibodies. Other agents, such as migratory inhibition factor (MIF), are produced in response to a specific stimulus by an immune cell population but are themselves relatively nonspecific (e.g., Kay, 1971). Only rarely has it proved possible to isolate and characterize these agents, and our knowledge of which cell produces which agent under what circumstances is rudimentary. More germane is the realization that many of the humoral products of lymphocytes have been demonstrated *in vitro* and we are profoundly uncertain of their significance in the intact animal; however, it seems reasonable to suppose that many of them will be found to be associated with autoregulation of the lymphoid system.

The thymus hormone constitutes a special case. The initial discovery that the thymus was in some way responsible for regulating the development of the lymphoid system—and thereby immunological capacity—was followed by a period of inquiry into how this effect was brought about. On the one hand evidence for the existence and significance of T cells accumulated, while on the other hand various extracts of thymus tissue and thymus grafts encapsulated in Millipore chambers were found to have effects of various degree on the lymphoid system (e.g., Davies, 1969). There came to be little doubt that a differentiational effect is exerted within the thymus by epithelial cells on lymphoid cell precursors, but the question remained (and still does) as to whether similar activities ever take place in lymphoid tissues outside the thymus. Perhaps the most interesting aspect of all this work has been the accumulation of evidence that extracts of lymphoid tissue, particularly thymus cells and materials diffusing from encapsulated lumps of more or less moribund thymus tissue, can have an appreciable augmentary effect on the lymphoid system (Davies, 1969). Earlier workers supposed that this effect was exerted on (in the present jargon) B cells or T-cell precursors; latterly it has become fashionable to suppose that it is on T cells—a sort of post-thymic maturation. It has been tentatively suggested that endotoxin-like materials could be responsible in certain instances for these influences, but more recent studies implicate a rather simpler low molecular weight peptide (Trainin and Small, 1970). Whatever the truth of the matter may be, it has become clear that various endotoxins can have very considerable stimulatory effects on the lymphoid system. But it remains to be seen whether these extrinsic agents are in any way related to similar materials produced as part of an autoregulatory mechanism within the lymphoid system.

It has been suggested that tissue regulation is mediated in part by chalones which can act as mitotic inhibitors. A specific lymphocyte chalone has been claimed (Bullough and Lawrence, 1970), but it remains to be seen whether chalones are in any way cognate with the various other humoral products of lymphocytes. Whatever the outcome of these various preliminary investigations, it is patent that the study of autoregulation within the lymphoid system is about to begin.

INTERNAL ENVIRONMENTAL FACTORS

Endocrine Status

It is well known that adrenocortical steroid hormones affect the lymphoid system, but what is not so certain is whether the effects are on B or T cells and whether they are reversible. In the past, the assumption has often been made that lymphocytes are lysed by steroid hormones, but these conclusions were all too frequently derived from experiments in which grossly unphysiological amounts of hormone had been used. These uncertainties should be resolved without too much difficulty by experiments in which animals with defined T (and perhaps B) cells are subjected to manipulations such as adrenalectomy which will affect their endocrine functions.

A whole new field of physiology lies here. From a more fundamental view it has already been shown that the development of the lymphoid system *ab initio* can be grossly affected by the levels of growth hormone (Baroni *et al.*, 1969; Pierpaoli and Sorkin, 1968). What is not established is whether pituitary hormone levels have any direct effect on the maintenance of normality in the adult lymphoid system.

Gut Flora

We do not presently know what effect the presence of a gut flora has on the T- and B-cell populations. Descriptively, it is apparent that the entire gut-associated lymphoid tissue of germ-free mice is less well developed than in conventional animals (Bauer, 1968). There is also a tendency for low peripheral blood lymphocyte counts and low immunoglobulin levels in germ-free rodents (Wostmann *et al.*, 1970). It is not clear at present whether these relative deficiencies relate to the T-cell or B-cell arms of the lymphoid system: development of the thymus is ostensibly normal in germ-free mice and the "thymus-dependent areas" are well stocked with cells, so that what evidence there is hints indirectly at a lack of B cells, a nuance happily in accord with the hypothesis expressed previously that B-cell amplification takes place in germinal centers.

EXTERNAL ENVIRONMENTAL FACTORS

Very many materials are administered to human beings which have effects on the lymphoid system. In some instances, as with immunosuppressants, the effects are intentional; in other cases, for example, in the chemotherapy of cancer, alteration of the lymphoid system is a more or less undesirable side effect. In only few instances can the precise target of immunosuppressive agents be specified, and for this reason the usage of such drugs is somewhat empirical. It is to be hoped that analytic studies of the effect of drugs on the lymphoid system will help to reduce this uncertainty. However, the most important class of extrinsic factors in relation to the lymphoid system is the various microorganisms and parasites, all of which in some way excite immunological responses by virtue of their antigenicity. Initially, the practice of immunology consisted largely of accumulation of *in vitro* tests for the measurement of the response to these invading organisms, and as a subsidiary benefit diagnostic antisera emerged which could be used to classify the organisms themselves. Slowly the emphasis is changing and more attention is being paid to the number and kinds of cells which participate in the reactions to antigenic materials and to host factors. The more sophisticated immunological approaches have aimed at simplification of antigenic materials, but many investigators have preferred to continue with the study of the responses to what have, colorfully, been called barnyard antigens. It is the responses to such materials which have provided us with the bulk of our information about the reaction modes of B and T cells in experimental animals. This is perhaps not inappropriate as many of the tests of the functional capacities of the lymphoid system in man relate to such antigens.

SOME HUMAN IMPLICATIONS

How far can these experimental models of lymphocyte systems be applied to man? As we have already pointed out, their complexity and artificiality have come under sharp attack (Burnet, 1970), and there is an obvious need to justify their wider relevance in clinical medicine. The change from mouse to man does, however, necessitate a considerable change in approach. The evidence for the existence of B- and T-cell systems in man is almost entirely inferential at the present time, and we therefore have to rely on indirect information relating to functional activity of the lymphoid system rather than on direct information concerned with B and T cells themselves. The major problem that arises here is the uncertainty surrounding the functional relationship between B and T cells. Some investigators dissociate B- and T-cell systems and regard them as independent entities, with B cells concerned with antibody responses and T cells concerned with cellular immune reactions of the delayed hypersensitivity type. Others believe that some interaction between the two systems is usually necessary for the full expression of the immune response, irrespective of whether that response is cellular or humoral. One consequence of this latter view is that it is (perhaps) no longer accurate to regard immune reactions as exclusively humoral or exclusively cellular. There is growing evidence that many allergens—tissue allografts, bacteria, viruses, tumors, skin-sensitizing agents—many evoke both humoral and cell-mediated immune responses. One type of immune reaction predominates, but the other can be demonstrated and the normal balance between them may be disturbed with profound effects on the host. This is particularly true of the immune responses to malignant cell populations, in which the presence of enhancing or blocking antibodies has been postulated to prevent cytotoxic effector cell attack on growing tumor cell masses (e.g., Hellström *et al.*, 1971).

The next problem is a more practical one. Although there are several immune reactions which can be used as more or less appropriate measures of T-cell and B-cell function in man, these reactions are not always deployed in the most appropriate fashion. In the case of humoral antibody formation, total antibody levels on their own may not be particularly revealing, and it is often desirable to test both primary and secondary immune responses, following (wherever possible) the whole course of the antibody response and determining the classes of immunoglobulins which are formed. Cellular immune reactions are more difficult to test, but it is expedient to examine both established and new delayed hypersensitivity responses, using a number of different allergens. Negative results may sometimes be due to depression rather than complete suppression, and a positive response may be elicited if the dose of allergen is increased and the time of the test prolonged. The assessment of PHA transformation *in vitro* needs particular care. Like delayed hypersensitivity reactions, the response to PHA may be slowed rather than absent, and impaired transformation may be due to factors other than an intrinsic lymphocyte defect. These include inhibitory factors circulating in the plasma, intercurrent viral infections, and the stress associated with surgery.

Many of these difficulties will be circumvented when reliable methods for the direct identification of B and T cells in man are devised. Three methods are available, but none of them has yet been fully exploited. In the exceptional circumstances where an athymic patient with the DiGeorge syndrome receives a thymus graft, the graft may be obtained from a donor of the opposite sex to the recipient; the sex chromosomes in these circumstances act as a convenient marker for recognizing donor T cells. Secondly, there is growing evidence from experimental studies that circulating blood lymphocytes which transform *in vitro* in the presence of PHA may be thymus-derived. Thirdly, it now seems probable that human thymus cells may carry an antigen similar to the θ and TL antigens described in T cells in mice (Yata et al., 1970).

The number and variety of clinical conditions which lend themselves to discussion in this section are extensive. Seemingly commonplace diseases such as measles may provide valuable insights into lymphocyte systems, a point illustrated by Burnet's (1970) masterly appraisal of measles "as an index of immunological function." We shall confine ourselves here to two broad groups of conditions in which the lymphoid system is either congenitally defective— the congenital immune deficiency states—or is neoplastic. And the discussion will deliberately have to be confined to a few selected aspects.

THE CONGENITAL IMMUNE DEFICIENCY STATES

These rare conditions, aptly described by Good and his colleagues as experiments of nature, have provided valuable clues to the components of the normal immune system in man (Good et al., 1962; Soothill, 1968; Gabrielson et al., 1969). Their importance is out of all proportion to their incidence. For purposes of discussion they may be divided into three major groups according to whether the immunological defect mainly affects humoral immunity, or cellular immunity, or is a combined abnormality involving both classes of the immune response to an approximately equal degree.

The first group is illustrated by the condition of sex-linked (Bruton) hypogammaglobulinemia. These patients have low levels of all three classes of immunoglobulins. Their antibacterial immunity is defective and they carry a high risk of bacterial infections, but their antiviral immunity, despite the absence of specific antibody, is ostensibly normal. This paradox is explained by the fact that cellular immune responses are for the most part intact. Delayed hypersensitivity reactions are readily elicited, and PHA transformation is normal (Marshall et al., 1970). The morphological findings in the lymphoid tissues fall into line with the immunological features: a general scarcity of lymphocytes, no plasma cells, and no follicles. The pharyngeal lymphoid tissues and Peyer's patches are extremely small. The thymus is usually normal, and thymus-dependent zones in the peripheral lymphoid tissues are intact (Peterson et al., 1965; Gabrielson et al., 1969).

There is no question that the major defect in children with congenital (Bruton) hypogammaglobulinemia involves the humoral side of the immune response, but there are certain anomalies which still require explanation. In particular, the defects in immunoglobulin synthesis may show a number of variations (Soothill, 1968). Production of serum immunoglobulins by individual patients often varies quite considerably when followed serially. Some patients have normal levels of one or more immunoglobulins—for instance, IgA and IgM—but grossly deficient levels of IgG. Other patients may show raised levels of IgM, though much of this appears to be functionally defective. Secondly, some patients with Bruton hypogammaglobulinemia have impaired skin homograft reactions (Good et al., 1962), a finding which is not easy to explain if the disease is characterized as an immunological defect confined exclusively to humoral immune mechanisms.

The second group of congenital immune deficiency disorders is illustrated by the DiGeorge syndrome, commonly regarded as a congenital absence of the thymus and parathyroid glands, probably due to anomalies in the early development of the third and fourth pharyngeal pouches. Patients have grossly defective cellular immune reactions, manifested by an inability to develop delayed hypersensitivity responses to a variety of bacterial, viral, and fungal proteins and to chemicals such as dinitrofluorobenzene (DNFB); impaired or absent rejection of skin homografts; and a failure of the blood lymphocytes to transform in vitro in the presence of PHA. By contrast, immunoglobulin levels are normal and antibody formation is commonly regarded as intact, or, at most, slightly depressed. Morphological studies show that the lymphoid tissues contain follicles and plasma cells, but the thymus-dependent zones are strikingly hypocellular. It should, however, be noted that some investigators now consider that humoral immune function in these patients may sometimes be more severely impaired than was formerly believed, a view which is discussed in detail a little later on. The DiGeorge syndrome is an obvious situation where thymus grafting may be considered as a therapeutic measure for restoring immune competence. At least two patients have now been treated in this way (August et al., 1968, 1970; Cleveland et al., 1968). Thymus grafting restored cell-mediated immune reactions, and this restoration was quickly established, complete, and seemingly permanent. Patients soon developed delayed hypersensitivity reactions to a variety of sensitizing agents, and the circulating lymphocytes responded normally to PHA in vitro.

Two aspects of the DiGeorge syndrome are worth considering in more detail—the question of impaired humoral immunity in this disease, and some of the wider implications of the consequences of thymus grafting.

Discussing the role of the thymus in humoral immunity, Lischner and DiGeorge (1969) have suggested that depression of antibody formation has been underestimated in thymic aplasia. They consider that complete absence of the thymus is associated with severe impairment of antibody formation, and they propose that patients with the DiGeorge syndrome in whom humoral immunity is largely intact may have had incomplete defects and "harbored small thymic remnants which were adequate to support some but not all immune functions." This conclusion is based largely on clinical inferences. Lischner and DiGeorge also point out that the presence of plasma cells in the lymphoid tissues can be interpreted in a number of ways. Antibody production need not be initiated solely by specifically activated antigen-sensitive cells; nonspecific stimuli may also operate, and possibly provide an explanation for the formation of defective immunoglobulins with no discernible antibody activity. The effects of thymectomy on antibody formation in experimental animals are also somewhat confusing. But it is probably fair to say that the primary and secondary antibody responses to many antigens are below normal after thymectomy, that the extent of the subnormal responses varies markedly, that there may be a particular deficiency in the formation of 7S-immunoglobulins, and that a few antigens (e.g., pneumococcal polysaccharide) evoke an antibody response which is seemingly independent of thymic function.

The second topic is the remarkable speed with which cell-mediated immunity is established in children with the DiGeorge syndrome when they are given a thymus graft (August et al., 1968, 1970; Cleveland et al., 1968). Delayed hypersensitivity reactions have been demonstrated within 2 weeks of thymus grafting, and a normal response of blood lymphocytes to PHA is found after only 4 days. In the patients so far studied, the cells which transformed in the presence of PHA have been *host* lymphocytes and there is no evidence that the donor thymus graft is a significant source of dividing cells. Two explanations come to mind for the mode of action of thymus grafts in these circumstances: the effects may be due to thymic hormone or perhaps to interaction between host lymphocytes and reticular cells in the donor thymus. The weight of evidence suggests that the lymphoid system in the DiGeorge syndrome is able to recognize and process many antigens but there is a failure in effector mechanisms; it is this failure which is repaired after thymus grafting.

The third category of combined deficiency syndromes comprises conditions where there is a gross defect of both humoral and cell-mediated processes. Three of these syndromes will serve to illustrate some of the features of the group. The most severe type of combined deficiency is found in reticular dysgenesis, characterized by a total developmental failure of all lymphoid cells (Soothill, 1968). Only three examples have been described, two in twins, and all these children died soon after birth. More information is available from another severe combined defect—lymphopenic (Swiss) hypogammaglobulinemia. There is almost complete aplasia of lymphocytes in the lymph nodes, spleen, and gastrointestinal tract in this condition, and there are no plasma cells. The thymus is minute and consists of little more than an epithelial anlage. Immunological failure is complete, and affected children rarely survive after 1 year. A less extreme combined deficiency is found in ataxia-telangiectasia. Both the morphological and immunological changes in this condition are variable (Peterson et al., 1965). Lymphocytes are usually reduced in the lymphoid tissues; plasma cells may either be absent or present in near normal numbers. The thymus contains well-developed epithelial and stromal components but few lymphocytes. Certain specific features of ataxia-telangiectasia are of interest: levels of circulating lymphocytes in the blood are normal, and the most usual immunoglobulin deficiency is a seemingly selective impairment of IgA synthesis. Susceptibility to fatal virus infection is less than in children with lymphopenic hypogammaglobulinemia: quite long survivals have been recorded, though some patients show progressive deterioration. There is evidence to suggest that patients with ataxia-telangiectasia who survive for a number of years may have an increased susceptibility to lymphoma (Peterson *et al.*, 1965). The number of cases is extremely small, but the implications are of great interest from the point of view of thymic function and immunological surveillance.

Certain general observations may be noted at this stage.

1. The clinical features of the congenital immune deficiency states have now been established in detail. The basic features of the various syndromes may, however, be modified by complicating factors due to chronic infection and malnutrition, and there may be spontaneous improvements and relapses. The range of possible defects and their combinations is extremely large (Soothill, 1968), and it is likely that many new variants will be described in the future. It seems reasonable to regard these conditions as part of a continuous spectrum, a view which emphasizes the need for a broad-based classification with the minimum of artificial subdivisions.

2. It is suggested that the present category of combined immune deficiencies (e.g., Swiss lymphopenic hypogammaglobulinemia and ataxia-telangiectasia) may need to be redefined. There is growing evidence that in most of the congenital immune deficiency syndromes cellular and humoral immunity are both impaired, though usually unequally. Defective cellular immunity predominates in some syndromes, defective humoral immunity predominates in others, and in a few conditions the defects may be equally severe; "pure" defects confined to one class of immune response are difficult to find. These observations lend support to the view that cellular and humoral immune reactions are not wholly independent and that, in most instances, some interaction between the two systems is necessary for the full expression of a particular immune response.

3. It is difficult to take the argument further and consider the specific activities of B and T cells in these syndromes since direct evidence relating to the function of B and T cells is hard to come by. Experimental findings indicate that B cells are concerned with antibody formation (Mitchell and Miller, 1968), and there is some evidence that T cells are directly concerned with cell-mediated immune responses (Miller and Brunner, 1970), but no such information is yet available for man.

LYMPHOID NEOPLASIA

The immunological changes associated with certain leukemias and lymphomas have been investigated intensively over the last decade. Initially regarded as a consequence of treatment by irradiation and cytotoxic drugs, it is now clear that the immune defects are an intrinsic part of the diseases concerned. The two conditions which have received particular attention are chronic lymphocytic leukemia and Hodgkin's disease, and it has become apparent that their immunological abnormalities differ in several fundamental respects.

Chronic lymphocytic leukemia is commonly regarded as a disease of immunologically incompetent lymphocytes, the leukemic cells accumulating progressively at the expense of a diminishing population of functionally normal lymphocytes (Dameshek, 1967). The brunt of the immune deficiency falls on that part of the immune system concerned with antibody responses. Total γ-globulin levels are low, especially during the later stages of the disease (Fairley and Scott, 1961). Individual antibody levels are below par in both primary and secondary responses (Cone and Uhr, 1964), and there is some evidence (see Harris and Sinkovics, 1970) that the induction time for IgM synthesis is delayed and that the usual IgM→IgG sequence is prolonged. Cellular immune function is better preserved: delayed hypersensitivity reactions to previously encountered antigens are usually intact, though the response to new sensitizing agents, such as 2,4-dinitrochlorobenzene (DNCB) is sometimes impaired or absent (Cone and Uhr, 1964). Rejection of skin homografts may be impaired (Miller et al., 1961). Patients with chronic lymphocytic leukemia are notoriously prone to bacterial and viral superinfections, and they can develop violent reactions to seemingly trivial incidents such as a mosquito bite or smallpox vaccination. There is also an increased incidence of autoimmune disease, principally autoimmune hemolytic anemia, thrombocytopenic purpura, and systemic lupus erythematosus.

As a result of these general findings, it has been proposed that chronic lymphocytic leukemia is a disease primarily affecting the thymus-independent B lymphocytes (Miller, 1967, 1968). Direct proof of the origin of these presumptive B cells is lacking, but some suggestive evidence has come from studies on the cells themselves. Many investigators have shown that most of the circulating lymphocytes in chronic lymphocytic leukemia do not transform in the presence of PHA; this failure is due to an intrinsic defect in the cell and not to some factor in the plasma. Since the evidence presently available suggests that in normal individuals it is mainly T cells that respond to PHA, the results of PHA transformation from the leukemic patients indicate that their peripheral blood lymphocytes comprise two different populations—a large group of nonresponding cells and a minority of PHA-sensitive cells. The nonresponding cells are perhaps B cells which (by other criteria) are abnormal and comprise the leukemic population; the responding cells are probably normal T cells. It is interesting that thoracic duct lymphocytes in chronic lymphocytic leukemia respond normally to PHA (Harris and Sinkovics, 1970), suggesting that PHA-refractory cells are confined to the blood vascular compartment. There is evidence from radioisotope studies that the leukemic lymphocytes in chronic lymphocytic leukemia are unable to leave the circulation (Stryckmans et al., 1968), and the existence of some kind of block at the postcapillary venules has been postulated. There is no obvious defect in the venules themselves, and Vincent and Gunz (1970) have proposed a membrane abnormality in the leukemic lymphocytes themselves. Gesner et al., (1969) have shown that the passage of lymphocytes through postcapillary venules may be modified by pretreatment with enzymes active against components of the lymphocyte membranes, and it is thus possible that a failure to respond to PHA and a failure to traverse the postcapillary venule may be linked through abnormalities in the cell surface.

It would seem at the present time that the immune deficiency in chronic lymphocytic leukemia chiefly affects humoral aspects of the immune response. Some investigators have seen similarities among the immune abnormalities in chronic lymphocytic leukemia, multiple myeloma, and sex-linked (Bruton) hypogammaglobulinemia (Miller, 1967, 1968; Aisenberg, 1966). But chronic lymphocytic leukemia appears to stand out in two respects: (1) the abnormal lymphocyte response to PHA *in vitro* and (2) the somewhat greater impairment of cellular immune function. The basic nature of the immune defects in chronic lymphocytic leukemia is still obscure and so is the relation of these defects to the underlying disease.

HODGKIN'S DISEASE

The immunological changes in Hodgkin's disease are more difficult to appraise, and the disease as a whole continues to bristle with unsolved problems. In contrast to chronic lymphocytic leukemia, there is no single distinguishing cell type, but there can be no doubt as to the central role of the lymphocyte in this disease. Recognition of this fact is perhaps the principal *raison d'être* of the recent histological classification of the disease which has established, among other things, the important clinical implications of lymphocyte predominance and lymphocyte depletion in affected lymphoid tissues (Lukes and Butler, 1966; Keller et al., 1968). Difficulties in interpreting the pleomorphic tissue response in Hodgkin's disease still remain, of course, and various ingenious theories have been put forward. Of particular interest is the view expressed by D. G. Miller (1967, 1968) that the morphological changes are essentially those of "an uncontrolled, self-perpetuating, malignant delayed hypersensitivity reaction," an interpretation which emphasizes that the immunological changes are a cardinal feature of the disease process rather than an exotic by-product of it. It has been recognized for several years that some of the clinical characteristics of Hodgkin's disease—wasting, anemia, and fever —are reminiscent of a graft *vs.* host reaction (Kaplan and Smithers, 1959; Smithers, 1967), and this leads one to examine the possibility that Hodgkin's disease is basically a disease of the part of the immune system concerned with cellular immunity, particularly involving T cells.

There is now abundant evidence that the immunological defects in Hodgkin's disease principally affect cell-mediated immunity. This is shown most convincingly by cutaneous anergy to bacterial, viral, fungal, and protozoal proteins, a defect which contributes to the increased incidence of superinfection by bacteria and other pathogens during the later stages of the disease. In many instances, anergy can be demonstrated *early* in patients in good clinical condition with localized disease and normal levels of circulating lymphocytes in the blood (Aisenberg, 1966). It is worth noting, though, that delayed hypersensitivity reactions in Hodgkin's disease are sometimes impaired rather than wholly suppressed at this stage; positive results may be produced if the dose of sensitizing agent is increased and/or the period of observation is prolonged. Patients are usually anergic to "new" sensitizing substances such as DNCB. Rejection of skin homografts is delayed or absent in patients with active disease, but homograft reactions during the early stages of Hodgkin's disease have not been described. The effects of PHA on lymphocytes *in vitro* are difficult to assess. Transformation is reduced in active disease, but both plasma and cellular defects may be responsible. The results of different studies are often contradictory, and the recent serial investigation of Jackson *et al.* (1970) is particularly valuable. These workers showed that the response was usually normal in localized Hodgkin's disease; it fell as the disease spread (probably independent of the peripheral lymphocytopenia) but tended to improve during periods of clinical remission. These results are not easy to interpret: if it is accepted that PHA transformation gives a reasonable measure of circulating T cells, a somewhat anomalous situation is found in early Hodgkin's disease, where seemingly normal numbers of T cells are present despite a definite impairment of delayed hypersensitivity as shown by cutaneous anergy to a number of sensitizing proteins. Lymphocyte transfer reactions have given interesting results in Hodgkin's disease: (1) lymphocytes from patients evoke a subnormal skin response in normal recipients, and (2) lymphocytes both from patients with Hodgkin's disease and from normal individuals produce equally poor responses when injected into a recipient with Hodgkin's disease (Aisenberg, 1965). Lastly, passive transfer of tuberculin sensitivity from normal subjects into patients with Hodgkin's disease, by means of donor leukocytes, has proved virtually impossible (Müftüoğlu and Balkuv, 1967). There is no intrinsic abnormality of the skin in Hodgkin's disease, and these findings point to at least two abnormalities—defective effector cells and perhaps a circulating inhibitory factor which interferes with the activities of normal lymphocytes.

Changes in humoral immune function in Hodgkin's disease are difficult to appraise from the literature. There is no doubt that such changes occur late and are overshadowed by the profound alterations in cellular immunity. Harris and Sinkovics (1970) suggest that primary antibody responses may be specifically impaired, and Aisenberg (1966) emphasizes the need to look at more subtle aspects of the process such as the evolution of the antibody response and the switchover from IgM to IgG production; there is perhaps a tendency to underestimate the changes in humoral immunity in this disease.

The immunological changes found in chronic lymphocytic leukemia and Hodgkin's disease cannot yet be satisfactorily interpreted, but a few general conclusions may be drawn.

1. In chronic lymphocytic leukemia, immunological defects tend to occur in the later stages of the disease. Abnormalities in humoral immunity predominate. Defects in cell-mediated immune processes are less common and less severe, but it is probably an oversimplification to regard the immune abnormalities in chronic lymphocytic leukemia as being *confined* to humoral antibody responses. It may eventually be established that it is B cells which are principally affected in chronic lymphocytic leukemia, with some minor damage to the T cell population—a situation which suggests a measure of interdependence between the B- and T-cell systems.

2. In Hodgkin's disease, the immune defect occurs early and consists predominantly of impaired cellular immunity. Abnormal humoral antibody responses are less marked and appear late. The immunological defects of Hodgkin's disease and chronic lymphocytic leukemia can be regarded as mirror images, but it is emphasized that there is some abnormality of humoral immunity in Hodgkin's disease and some abnormality of cell-mediated immunity in chronic lymphocytic leukemia. The defect in Hodgkin's disease may eventually be shown to fall predominantly (but not exclusively) on T cells. It is, however, clear that other noncellular factors are present in Hodgkin's disease which affect parameters of immune function such as lymphocyte transfer tests, the passive transfer of delayed hypersensitivity, and PHA transformation. The contribution of these factors to the immunological changes associated with Hodgkin's disease is unknown.

3. The previous discussion has had to ignore completely several fundamental points relating to both diseases. Why, in particular, do chronic lymphocytic leukemia and Hodgkin's disease persist and progress? Is this due to

persistence of antigen (e.g., a virus)? Or the emergence of a forbidden clone of B or T cells? Or a failure of feedback mechanisms?

This account of lymphocyte systems in mouse and man has been deliberately speculative. Some, perhaps most, of it will undoubtedly need to be modified in the light of fresh experimental findings over the next few years. Prediction of future trends of investigations is rash, but it seems reasonable to suppose that there will be continuing efforts to characterize the B- and T-cell systems of lymphocytes more closely in terms of organization, interaction, and function. The potential advantages which would accrue to clinical medicine from a greater knowledge of these lymphocyte systems are so tremendous that they must surely continue to stimulate basic investigations in this field.

REFERENCES

Ada, G. L., Parrish, C. R., Nossal, G. J. V., and Abbot, A., 1967. The tissue localization, immunogenic, and tolerance-inducing properties of antigens and antigen-fragments. *Cold Spring Harbor Symp. Quant. Biol. (Antibodies).* 32:381.

Aisenberg, A. C., 1965. Studies of lymphocyte transfer reactions in Hodgkin's disease. *J. Clin. Invest.* 44:555.

Aisenberg, A. C., 1966. Immunologic status of Hodgkin's disease. *Cancer* (New York), 19:385.

Askonas, B. A., Williamson, A. R., and Wright, B. E. G., 1970. Selection of a single antibody-forming cell clone and its propagation in syngeneic mice. *Proc. Natl. Acad. Sci.* 67:1398.

August, C. S., Rosen, F. S., Filler, R. M., Janeway, C. A., Markowski, B., and Kay, H. E. M., 1968. Implantation of a foetal thymus, restoring immunological competence in a patient with thymic aplasia (DiGeorge's syndrome). *Lancet* ii:1210.

August, C. S., Berkel, A. I., Levey, R. H., Rosen, F. S., and Kay, H. E. M., 1970. Establishment of immunological competence in a child with congenital thymic aplasia by a graft of fetal thymus. *Lancet* i: 1080.

Bach, J.-F., Muller, J.-Y., and Dardenne, M., 1970. *In vivo* specific antigen recognition by rosette forming cells. *Nature* (London) 227:1251.

Baroni, C. D., Fabris, N., and Bertoli, G., 1969. Effects of hormones on development and function of lymphoid tissues. Synergistic action of thyroxin and somatotropic hormone in pituitary dwarf mice. *Immunology* 17:303.

Bauer, H., 1968. Defence mechanisms in germ-free animals. Part II. Cellular defence mechanisms. In Coates, M. E., ed., *The Germ-Free Animal in Research,* Academic Press, New York, p. 210.

Borum, K., 1968. Pattern of cell production and cell migration in mouse thymus studied by autoradiography. *Scand. J. Haematol.* 5:339.

Boyse, E. A., Lance, E. M., Carswell, E. A., Cooper, S., and Old, L. J., 1970. Rejection of skin allografts by radiation chimaeras: Selective gene action in the specification of cell surface structure. *Nature* (London) 227:901.

Brahim, F., and Osmond, D. G., 1970. Migration of bone-marrow lymphocytes demonstrated by selective bone marrow labelling with thymidine-H[3]. *Anat. Rec.* 168:139.

Bullough, W. S., and Lawrence, E. B., 1970. The lymphocytic chalone and its antimitotic action on a mouse lymphoma *in vitro. Europ. J. Cancer* 6:525.

Burnet, M., 1970. *Immunological Surveillance,* Pergamon Press, Australia.

Claman, H. N., Chaperon, E. A., and Triplett, R. F., 1966. Immunocompetence of transferred thymus-marrow cell combinations. *J. Immunol.* 97:828.

Cleveland, W. W., Fogel, B. J., Brown, W. T., and Kay, H. E. M., 1968. Foetal thymic transplant in a case of DiGeorge syndrome. *Lancet* ii:1211.

Cone, L., and Uhr, J. W., 1964. Immunological deficiency disorders associated with chronic lymphocytic leukaemia and multiple myeloma. *J. Clin. Invest.* 43:2241.

Cottier, H., Hess, M. W., and Stoner, R. D., 1967. Summary and closing remarks. In Cottier, H., Odartchenko, N., Schindler, R., and Congdon, C. C., eds., *Germinal Centers in Immune Responses*, Springer-Verlag, Berlin, Heidelberg, New York, p. 460.

Dameshek, W., 1967. Chronic lymphocytic leukemia—an accumulative disease of immunologically incompetent lymphocytes. *Blood* 29:566.

Davies, A. J. S., 1969. The thymus humoral factor under scrutiny. *Agents and Actions* 1:1.

Davies, A. J. S., Leuchars, E., Wallis, V., and Koller, P. C., 1966. The mitotic response of thymus-derived cells to antigenic stimulus. *Transplantation* 4:438.

Davies, A. J. S., Leuchars, E., Wallis, V., Marchant, R., and Elliott, E. V., 1967. The failure of thymus-derived cells to produce antibody. *Transplantation* 5:222.

Davies, A. J. S., Carter, R. L., Leuchars, E., and Wallis, V., 1969a. The morphology of immune reactions in normal, thymectomized and reconstituted mice. II. The response to oxazolone. *Immunology* 17:111.

Davies, A. J. S., Carter, R. L., Leuchars, E., Wallis, V., and Koller, P. C., 1969b. The morphology of immune reactions in normal, thymectomized and reconstituted mice. I. The response to sheep erythrocytes. *Immunology* 16:57.

Davies, A. J. S., Leuchars, E., Wallis, V., and Doenhoff, M. J., 1971. A system for lymphocytes in the mouse. *Proc. Roy. Soc. Lond. B* 176:369.

Doenhoff, M. J., and Davies, A. J. S., 1971. Reconstitution of the "T" cell pool following irradiation of mice. *Cell. Immunol.* 2:82.

Ernström, U., and Sandberg, G., 1970. Quantitative relationship between release and intrathymic death of lymphocytes. *Acta Pathol. Microbiol. Scand., Sect. A.,* 78:362.

Fairley, G. H., and Scott, R. B., 1961. Hypogammaglobulinaemia in chronic lymphocytic leukemia. *Brit. Med. J.* 2:920.

Florey, H., 1970. *General Pathology,* 4th ed., Lloyd-Luke (Medical Books) Ltd., London.

Ford, C. E., and Micklem, H. S., 1963. The thymus and lymph-nodes in radiation chimaeras. *Lancet* 1:359.

Ford, C. E., Hamerton, J. L., Barnes, D. W. H., and Loutit, J. F., 1956. Cytological identification of radiation-chimaeras. *Nature* (London), 177:452.

Ford, W. L., 1969. The immunological and migratory properties of the lymphocytes recirculating through the rat spleen. *Brit. J. Exptl. Pathol.* 50:257.

Gabrielson, A. E., Cooper, M. D., Peterson, R. D. A., and Good, R. A., 1969. The primary immunologic deficiency diseases. In Miescher, P. A., and Müller-Eberhard, H. J., eds., *Textbook of Immunopathology,* Vol. II, Grune and Stratton, New York, p. 385.

Gengozian, N., Urso, I. S., Congdon, C. C., Conger, A. D., and Makinodan, T., 1957. Thymus specificity in lethally irradiated mice treated with rat bone marrow. *Proc. Soc. Exptl. Biol. Med.* 96:714.

Gesner, B. M., Woodruff, J. J., and McCluskey, R. T., 1969. An autoradiographic study of the effects of neuraminidase or trypsin on transfused lymphocytes. *Am. J. Pathol.* 57:215.

Glick, B., Chang, T. S., and Jaap, R. G., 1956. The bursa of Fabricius and antibody production in the domestic fowl. *Poultry Sci.* 35:224.

Globerson, A., and Auerbach, R., 1966. Primary antibody response in organ cultures. *J. Exptl. Med.* 124:1001.

Good, R. A., Kelly, W. D., Rötstein, J., and Varco, R. L., 1962. Immunological deficiency diseases. Agammaglobulinemia, hypogammaglobulinemia, Hodgkin's disease, and sarcoidosis. *Progr. Allergy,* 6:187.

Gowans, J. L., 1959. The recirculation of lymphocytes from blood to lymph in the rat. *J. Physiol.* (London), 146:54.

Hall, J. G., and Morris, B., 1964. Effect of X-irradiation of the popliteal lymph-node on its output of lymphocytes and immunological responsiveness. *Lancet* 1:1077.

Hall, J. G., and Morris, B., 1965. The origin of the cells in the efferent lymph from a single lymph node. *J. Exptl. Med.* 121:901.

Hanna, M. G., Jr., Szakal, R. K., and Walburg, H. E., Jr., 1969. The relation of antigen and virus localization in the development and growth of germinal centers. In Fiore-Donati, L., and Hanna, M. G., eds., *Lymphatic Tissue and Germinal Centers in Immune Response,* Plenum Press, New York, p. 149.

Hannig, K., and Zeiller, K., 1969. Zur Auftrennung und Characterizierung immunkompetente Zellung mit Hilfe des Trägerfreien Ablenkungselectrophorese. *Z. Phys. Chem.* 350:467.

Harris, J. E., and Sinkovics, J. G., 1970. *The Immunology of Malignant Disease,* Henry Kingston, London.

Harris, T. N., Harris, S., and Farber, M. B., 1954. Transfer to X-irradiated rabbits of lymph node cells incubated *in vitro* with *Shigella paradysenteriae. Proc. Soc. Exptl. Biol. Med.* 86:549.

Hellström, I., Sjögren, H. O., Warner, G., and Hellström, K. E., 1971. Blocking of cell-mediated tumor immunity by sera from patients with growing neoplasms. *Internat. J. Cancer* 7:226.

Hewson, W., 1777. In Falconer, M., ed., *Experimental Inquiries into the Properties of the Blood,* T. Cadell, London, p. 85.

Hinrichsen, K., 1965. Zellteilungen und Zellwanderungen im Thymus der erwachsenen Maus. *Z. Zellforsch.* 68:427.

Hunter, R. L., Wissler, R. W., and Fitch, F. W., 1969. Studies on the kinetics and radiation sensitivity of dendritic macrophages. In Fiore-Donati, L., and Hanna, M. G., eds., *Lymphatic Tissue and Germinal Centers in Immune Response,* Plenum Press, New York, p. 101.

Jackson, S. M., Garrett, J. V., and Craig, A. W., 1970. Lymphocyte transformation changes during the clinical course of Hodgkin's disease. *Cancer* (New York), 25:843.

Jeejeebhoy, H. F., 1965. Immunological studies in the rat thymectomized in adult life. *Immunology* 9:417.

Jerne, N. K., and Nordin, A. A., 1963. Plaque formation in agar by single antibody-producing cells. *Science* 140:405.

Kaplan, H. S., and Smithers, D. W., 1959. Autoimmunity in man and homologous disease in mice in relation to the malignant lymphomas. *Lancet* ii:1.

Kay, H. E. M., 1971. Lymphocyte function. *Brit. J. Haematol.* 20:139.

Keller, A. R., Kaplan, H. S., Lukes, R. J., and Rappaport, H., 1968. Correlation of histopathology with other prognostic indicators in Hodgkin's disease. *Cancer* (New York), 22:487.

Köbberling, G., 1965. Autoradiographische Untersuchungen über Zellursprung und Zellwanderung in lymphatischen Organen fetaler und neugeborener Mäuse. *Z. Zellforsch.* 68:631.

Koller, P. C., Davies, A. J. S., Leuchars, E., and Wallis, V., 1966. Mitotic activity of two chromosomally marked populations of cells in an immune response. In *Germinal Centers in Immune Responses,* Springer-Verlag, Berlin, Heidelberg, New York, p. 157.

Lance, E. M., Cooper, S., and Boyse, E. A., 1971. Antigenic change and cell maturation in murine thymocytes. *Cell. Immunol.* 1:536.

Leuchars, E., Morgan, A., Davies, A. J. S., and Wallis, V. J., 1967. Thymus grafts in thymectomized and normal mice. *Nature* (London), **214**:801.

Lischner, H. W., and DiGeorge, A. M., 1969. Role of the thymus in humoral immunity. *Lancet* ii:1044.

Lukes, R. J., and Butler, J. J., 1966. The pathology and nomenclature of Hodgkin's disease. *Cancer Res.* **26**:1063.

Marchesi, V. T., and Gowans, J. L., 1964. The migration of lymphocytes through the endothelium of venules in lymph nodes in an electron microscope study. *Proc. Roy. Soc. Lond. B* **159**:283.

Marshall, W. C., Cope, W. A., Soothill, J. F., and Dudgeon, J. A., 1971. *In vitro* lymphocyte response in some immunity deficiency diseases and in intrauterine virus infections. *Proc. Roy. Soc. Med.* **63**:351.

Metcalf, D., 1965. Multiple thymus grafts in aged mice. *Nature* (London), **208**:87.

Metcalf, D., 1966. Recent results in cancer research. In *The Thymus: Its Role in Immune Responses, Leukemia Development and Carcinogenesis*, Springer-Verlag, Berlin, Heidelberg, New York.

Miller, D. G., 1967. Immunological deficiency and malignant lymphoma. *Cancer* (New York), **20**:579.

Miller, D. G., 1968. The immunologic capability of patients with lymphoma. *Cancer Res.* **28**:1441.

Miller, D. G., Lizardo, J. G., and Synderman, R. K., 1961. Homologous and heterologous skin transplantation in patients with lymphomatous disease. *J. Natl. Cancer Inst.* **26**:569.

Miller, J. F. A. P., 1965. Effect of thymectomy in adult mice on immunological responsiveness. *Nature* (London), **208**:1337.

Miller, J. F. A. P., and Brunner, K. T., 1970. Thymus-derived cells as killer cells in cell-mediated immunity. Third Internat. Congr. Transplantation Soc., The Hague, September 1970.

Miller, J. F. A. P., and Davies, A. J. S., 1964. Embryological development of the immune mechanism. *Ann. Rev. Med.* **15**:23.

Mishell, R. I., and Dutton, R. W., 1967. Immunization of dissociated spleen cell cultures from normal mice. *J. Exptl. Med.* **126**:423.

Mitchell, G. F., and Miller, J. F. A. P., 1968. Immunological activity of thymus and thoracic-duct lymphocytes. *Proc. Natl. Acad. Sci.* **59**:296.

Moore, M. A. S., and Owen, J. J. T., 1967. Stem-cell migration in developing myeloid and lymphoid systems. *Lancet* ii:658.

Morris, B., 1968. Migration intratissulaire des lymphocytes du mouton. *Nouv. Rev. Française Hématol.* **8**:525.

Müftüoğlu, A. U., and Balkuv, S., 1967. Passive transfer of tuberculin sensitivity to patients with Hodgkin's disease. *New Engl. J. Med.* **277**:126.

Nossal, G. J. V., and Gorrie, J., 1964. Studies of the emigration of thymic cells in young guinea pigs. In Good, R. A., and Gabrielson, A. E., eds., *The Thymus in Immunobiology*, Harper and Row, New York, p. 288.

Nowell, P. C., 1960. Phytohaemagglutinin: An initiator of mitosis in cultures of normal human leucocytes. *Cancer Res.* **20**:462.

Owen, J. J. T., and Raff, M. C., 1970. Studies on the differentiation of thymus-derived lymphocytes. *J. Exptl. Med.* **132**:1216.

Owen, J. J. T., and Ritter, M. A., 1969. Tissue interaction in the development of thymus lymphocytes. *J. Exptl. Med.* **129**:431.

Ozer, H., and Waksman, B. H., 1970. Appendix and γM antibody formation. IV. Synergism of appendix and bone marrow cells in early antibody response to sheep erythrocytes. *J. Immunol.* **105**:791.

Parrott, D. M. V., de Sousa, M. A. B., and East, J., 1966. Thymus-dependent areas in the lymphoid organs of neonatally thymectomized mice. *J. Exptl. Med.* **123**:191.

Peterson, R. D. H., Cooper, M. D., and Good, R. A., 1965. The pathogenesis of immunologic deficiency diseases. *Am. J. Med.* 38:579.

Pierpaoli, W., and Sorkin, E., 1968. Hormones and immunologic capacity. I. Effect of heterologous anti-growth hormone (ASTH) antiserum on thymus and peripheral lymphatic tissue in mice. Induction of a wasting syndrome. *J. Immunol.* 101:1036.

Raff, M. C., 1969. Theta isoantigen as a marker of thymus-derived lymphocytes in mice. *Nature* (London), 224:378.

Raff, M. C., 1971. Evidence for a subpopulation of mature lymphocytes within mouse thymus. *Nature* (London), 229:182.

Raff, M. C., and Wortis, H. H., 1970. Thymus dependent θ bearing cells in peripheral lymphoid tissues of mice. *Immunology* 18:931.

Raff, M. C., Nase, S., and Mitchison, N. A., 1971. Mouse specific bone marrow–derived lymphocyte antigen as a marker for thymus-independent lymphocytes. *Nature* (London), 230:50.

Raidt, D. J., Mishell, R. I., and Dutton, R. W., 1968. Cellular events in the immune response. Analysis and *in vitro* response of mouse spleen cell populations separated by differential flotation in albumin gradients. *J. Exptl. Med.* 128:681.

Reif, A. E., and Allen, J. M. V., 1964. The AKR thymic antigen and its distribution in leukemias and nervous tissues. *J. Exptl. Med.* 120:413.

Roitt, I. M., Greaves, M. F., Torrigiani, G., Brostoff, J., and Playfair, J. H. L., 1969. The cellular basis of immunological responses. A synthesis of some current views. *Lancet* 2:367.

Slonecker, C. E., Sordat, E., and Hess, M. W., 1969. Lymphatic drainage of thymic lymphocytes in mice. In Fiore-Donati, L., and Hanna, M. G., eds., *Lymphatic Tissue and Germinal Centers in Immune Response*, Plenum Press, New York, p. 125.

Smithers, D. W., 1967. Hodgkin's disease. *Brit. Med. J.* 2:263 and 337.

Soothill, J. F., 1968. Immune deficiency states. In Gell, P. G. H., and Coombs, R. R. A., eds., *Clinical Aspects of Immunology*, 2nd ed., Blackwell, Oxford, p. 540.

Stryckmans, P. A., Chanana, A. D., Cronkite, E. P., Greenberg, M. L., and Schiffer, L. M., 1968. Studies on lymphocytes. IX. The survival of autotransfused labelled lymphocytes in chronic lymphocytic leukemia. *Europ. J. Cancer* 4:241.

Taylor, R. B., 1965. Decay of immunological responsiveness after thymectomy in adult life. *Nature* (London), 208:1334.

Trainin, N., and Small, M., 1970. Studies on some physicochemical properties of a thymus humoral factor conferring immunocompetence on lymphoid cells. *J. Exptl. Med.* 132:885.

van Bekkum, D. W., and Vos, O., 1957. Immunological aspects of homo- and heterologous bone marrow transplantation in irradiated animals. *J. Cell Comp. Physiol.* 50: Suppl. 1, 139.

Vincent, P. C., and Gunz, F. W., 1970. Control of lymphocyte level in the blood. *Lancet* ii:342.

Warner, N. L., and Szenberg, A., 1964. Immunologic studies on hormonally bursectomized and surgically thymectomized chickens: Dissociation of immunologic responsiveness. In Good, R. A., and Gabrielson, A. E., eds., *The Thymus in Immunobiology*, Harper and Row, New York, p. 395.

Wigzell, H., and Andersson, B., 1969. Cell separation on antigen-coated columns. Eliminations of high rate antibody-forming cells and immunological memory cells. *J. Exptl. Med.* 129:23.

Wostmann, B. S., Pleasants, J. R., Bealmear, P., and Kincade, P. W., 1970. Serum proteins and lymphoid tissues in germ-free mice fed a chemically defined, water soluble, low molecular weight diet. *Immunology* 19:443.

Yata, J., Klein, G., Kobayashi, N., Furukawa, T., and Yanagisawa, M., 1970. Human thymus-lymphoid tissue antigen and its presence in leukemia and lymphoma. *Clin. Exptl. Immunol.* 7:781.

Yoffey, J. M., and Olson, I. A., 1966. Oligosynthetic and polysynthetic lymph nodes. In Yoffey, J. M., ed., *The Lymphocyte in Immunology and Haemopoiesis,* Edward Arnold Ltd., London, p. 358.

Zaalberg, O. B., 1964. A simple method for detecting single antibody-forming cells. *Nature* (London), 202:1231.

Chapter 2

A Developmental Approach to the Biological Basis for Antibody Diversity

Max D. Cooper,* Alexander R. Lawton,† and Paul W. Kincade‡
Spain Research Laboratories
Departments of Pediatrics and Microbiology
University of Alabama Medical Center
Birmingham, Alabama

INTRODUCTION

The emphasis in this discussion will be on early events in differentiation of antibody-producing cells, an area of immunology that is in its experimental infancy. Most of the available information on the antibody problem emerged from analyses of relatively mature cells of the plasma cell lineage and the end products they secrete. Several useful theories on the development of antibody heterogeneity taking into account the diversity and specificity of antibody molecules, the restrictions imposed by genetic and structural analyses, and the phenomenon of self-recognition have been proposed. However, the paucity of knowledge of the origin, identity, and characterization of pre-antibody forming cells has been a handicap in the struggle toward a final solution of this problem.

Since the discovery that antibody-producing cells are developmentally independent of the thymus line of lymphocytes mediating cellular immunity, considerable progress has been made in defining some of the earliest events in plasma cell differentiation. The chicken has been a favorite model for such

Supported by grants from the National Institutes of Health (AI-08345 and RR-05349) and The American Cancer Society.
* American Cancer Society Faculty Research Associate, Professor of Pediatrics, and Associate Professor of Microbiology.
† U.S.P.H.S. Special Postdoctoral Fellow (AI-42973).
‡ U.S.P.H.S. Predoctoral Fellow (GM-43118).

studies primarily because in this animal the site of induction of stem cells along plasma cell lines occurs in the bursa of Fabricius, an easily removable hindgut lymphoepithelial organ. It is our belief that this approach has already provided information relevant to the quest for understanding the mechanisms responsible for development of antibody diversity.

Results to be reviewed suggest that (1) immunoglobulin synthesis is initiated in cells within lymphoid follicles of the bursa; (2) onset of immunoglobulin synthesis appears to be a normal event in cellular differentiation rather than one that is dependent on the influences of exogenous antigens; (3) immunoglobulins produced by lymphoid cells in the bursa are secreted poorly, if at all, but may be incorporated into the cell membranes, where they fulfill the role of "recognition antibodies," as postulated in the clonal selection theory of Burnet; (4) IgG-producing cells are the progeny of IgM-producing cells; (5) the "switchover" in immunoglobulin classes within individual clones of cells occurs only, or primarily, within the bursa; and (6) once seeded from the bursa, lymphoid cells bearing "recognition antibodies" are committed in regard to class and specificity of the antibodies which they can make and secrete once stimulated by antigen. This line of reasoning and its supporting evidence argue that elucidation of the developmental basis for antibody diversity requires an understanding of the interrelationship between stem cells and the microenvironment in which plasma cell differentiation is initiated. Toward this end, a general theoretical framework is presented.

DEVELOPMENT OF THE BURSAL LINE OF CELLS IN CHICKENS

From their original location in the yolk sac, stem cells migrate to the bursa of Fabricius to begin differentiation along plasma cell lines. These cells have been characterized histologically by their large size, deeply basophilic cytoplasm, and an abundance of euchromatin. Cells of yolk sac origin are first detectable in the bursa, using chromosomal markers, on the thirteenth day of incubation, that is, 7 or 8 days before hatching (Moore and Owen, 1966). Even before the onset of this immigration to the bursa, foci of thickened epithelium can be found among the cells lining the luminal surface of the bursa (Fig. 1). The signals for budding of the epithelium are unknown, but the high alkaline phosphatase content of mesenchymal cells underneath these "epithelial buds" may play a role in this process (Ackerman and Knouff, 1964).

Within 24 hr after arrival of the yolk sac stem cells, lymphoid cells containing cytoplasmic μ- and light-chain antigenic determinants can be demonstrated in many of the developing bursal follicles (Kincade and Cooper, 1971). Over the next few days, the lymphoepithelial follicles enlarge and the

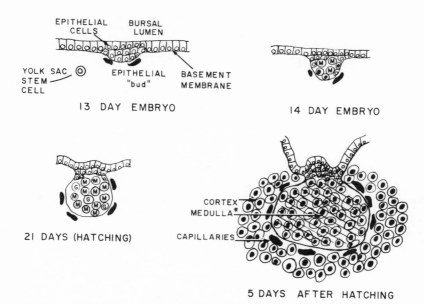

Figure 1. Schematic outline of the development of bursal follicles.*–Contiguous deposition of IgM and IgG, indicated by shading, is usually found in bursal follicles of birds at this age or beyond.

number of IgM-containing cells within them increases correspondingly. Although some of this population increase may be due to continued influx of stem cells, most is probably attributable to local cell replication. The average generation time of follicular cells at 15 days of embryonic life is 7-9 hr (Rubin, 1971). At any one time, an average of approximately 50% of the cells within individual follicles are engaged in DNA synthesis. All of these events occur in an environment relatively sheltered from exogenous antigens and at a time in embryonic life when IgM-containing cells are not detectable in the yolk sac, liver, intestine, spleen, or thymus. Furthermore, at this stage in development, IgM is not detectable in the circulation.

One week after the appearance of IgM-containing cells in bursal follicles, IgG-containing cells become demonstrable by immunofluorescent techniques. These cells are always observed within follicles already populated with IgM-containing cells. The emergence of IgG-containing cells in the bursa cannot be hastened by injection of several potent antigens or of adult plasma (Kincade and Cooper, 1971). These observations suggest that, in contrast to development of antibody-secreting cells in peripheral lymphoid tissues, immunoglobulin-containing cells in bursal follicles produce immunoglobulins as a normal event in differentiation and not under the influence of exogenous antigens. By use of *in vitro* incorporation of radiolabeled amino acids, developmental studies of chicken lymphoid tissues also show the bursa to be the first site of immunoglobulin synthesis (Thorbecke *et al.*, 1968).

The inducer substances which influence stem cells to begin their specialized differentiation within the bursal microenvironment are presently undefined. Such factors may come from the bursal lumen, since bursal lymphopoietic activity ceases when the organ is transplanted to sites where it is not connected to the intestinal lumen (Thompson and Cooper, 1971). The epithelium directly overlying lymphoid follicles of the bursa differs from other bursal epithelium in that it is specially adapted to transport substances from the lumen by the process of pinocytosis (Bockman and Cooper, 1971).

Bursal cells subsequently migrate to other areas of the body, where they respond to antigenic stimulation by cell division and maturation to become antibody-secreting cells. Identification of bursa-derived cells in extrabursal sites has been facilitated by study of the immune system in bursectomized birds. Peripheral development of the plasma cell line can be aborted or prevented entirely by (1) removal of the bursa on or before the seventeenth day of incubation (Cooper *et al.*, 1969), (2) chemical bursectomy produced by testosterone administration early in embryonic life (Warner *et al.*, 1969), or (3) bursectomy at hatching followed by near lethal whole-body exposure to X-rays (Cooper *et al.*, 1966a). Birds so treated lack lymphoid cells with the fine structural characteristics of bursal cells (Clawson *et al.*, 1967), germinal centers, and plasma cells; they are agammaglobulinemic as judged by (1) absence of detectable immunoglobulins in the circulation, (2) absence of detectable antibodies following repeated immunizations with potent antigens even when very sensitive antibody detection techniques are employed, (3) lack of detectable antigen-binding cells, and (4) lack of cells containing detectable amounts of cytoplasmic or membrane-bound immunoglobulins (Kincade *et al.*, 1971). On the other hand, germinal centers, plasma cells, and immunoglobulin synthesis can be restored in such birds by infusion of histocompatible bursal lymphoid cells from a newly hatched chick (Cooper *et al.*, 1966b), and selective migration of labeled bursal cells to germinal centers has been demonstrated using radioautographic techniques (Durkin *et al.*, 1971).

The developmental sequence of IgM followed by IgG is recapitulated in extrabursal sites (Kincade and Cooper, 1971; Thorbecke *et al.*, 1968). In chicken embryos commonly infected with vertically transmitted pathogens, cells containing detectable amounts of cytoplasmic IgM are occasionally encountered in peripheral sites during embryonic life; the earliest one found was located in the lamina propria of the intestine of a 17-day embryo, and by the nineteenth day a few were found in the spleen and thymus. On the other hand, IgG-containing cells have not been found in extrabursal sites until the fourth day after hatching. In chicks raised in conventional environments, rapid expansion of the IgM-containing population in the spleen begins around the third day after hatching; IgG-containing cells begin a similar expansion in numbers somewhere around the eighth day of life. As a consequence of this sequence of cell development, the rise of IgG levels in the circulation lags behind that of IgM by a significant interval (Van Meter et al., 1969). In striking contrast to the development of immunoglobulin-producing cells in the bursa, the development of antibody-producing cells in peripheral sites is clearly antigen-dependent (Kincade and Cooper, 1971; Thorbecke et al., 1968). For example, chicks uncontaminated with the usual pathogens transmitted from hen to egg, hatched into a germ-free environment, and given only sterile deionized water develop few, if any, detectable immunoglobulin-containing cells in extrabursal sites over a 5-day period after hatching (Kincade and Cooper, 1971).

In light of these observations, it is not surprising that bursal control of the sequential development of IgM synthesis followed by IgG synthesis in extrabursal sites can be demonstrated by removal of the bursa at different times during development. As mentioned earlier, agammaglobulinemic chicks can be produced by removal of the bursa on or before the seventeenth day of embryonic life. Bursectomy of 19-day embryos usually does not impair development of IgM-producing cells in extrabursal tissues but prevents or severely stunts subsequent development of IgG-producing cells. Removal of the bursa on the twenty-first day of incubation (the usual time of hatching) slows, but usually does not prevent, subsequent development of normal circulating levels of both IgM and IgG (Van Meter et al., 1969).

With this information in mind, it seemed logical to focus attention on the bursa in a search for additional clues to the basis for the developmental sequence of the two immunoglobulin classes. As mentioned before, fluorescent analysis of immunoglobulin-containing cells during development revealed that IgG-containing cells initially arose in bursal follicles already populated by IgM-containing cells. In sections of bursas from more mature chicks, the follicular distribution of fluorescence produced by antisera to IgG and IgM is superimposable except for a few follicles that appear to be populated only by IgM-containing cells. These observations suggested that cells containing both immunoglobulins might exist in bursal follicles. Analysis of the immunoglobulin content of single bursal cells provided support for this hypothesis; approximately 50% of bursal cells identified as IgG-containing cells by fluorescein-tagged antibodies could be subsequently stained by rhodamine-tagged antibodies specific for IgM (Kincade and Cooper, 1971). Similar analysis of spleen cells rarely revealed single cells containing both classes of immunoglobulins. These observations suggested that a "switchover" from IgM to IgG synthesis might occur within clones of lymphocytes in the bursa. To discriminate between this and other possibilities, purified goat antibodies to antigenic determinants of chicken μ chains were given intravenously to 13-day chick embryos. These birds were bursectomized at hatching in order to prevent recovery from the suppressive effects of the anti-μ antibodies. This treatment effectively suppressed or abolished IgM synthesis in experimental birds; IgG synthesis was suppressed as efficiently as IgM (Kincade et al., 1970). If sufficient amounts of anti-μ were given and followed by bursectomy at hatching, agammaglobulinemic chicks, normal in their capacity to reject skin allografts, could be produced with regularity. Morphologic evaluation of the bursas in anti-μ treated embryos provided evidence suggesting that selective elimination of IgM-containing cells had been achieved. Although other interpretations of these observations have been considered, it seems difficult to escape the conclusion that IgG-producing cells arise within the bursa from cells containing IgM.

Attention was then directed to the question of whether or not a "switchover" of IgM producers to IgG-producing cells could occur outside the bursa. Newly hatched chicks were subjected to bursectomy and then given injections of anti-μ antibodies; controls were treated similarly but received normal goat γ-globulin. Birds belonging to the anti-μ treated group were strikingly deficient in the ability to make IgM but produced amounts of IgG as high as those found in control birds (Kincade et al., 1970). The same question has been addressed by another experimental approach. Birds can be rendered selectively deficient in IgG-producing cells by removal of the bursa at an appropriate age in development. Immunoglobulin levels have been monitored for as long as 8 months in such birds; they produce supernormal levels of IgM but never repair their deficiency of IgG (unpublished observations), as would be expected if extrabursal IgM producers could switch, in significant numbers, to become IgG-producing cells. We conclude that such is not the case.

Before discussing our theoretical synthesis of these observations, some additional features of bursal lymphocytes will be reviewed. Near the time of hatching, a distinct mantle of lymphoid cells begins to develop around the bursal follicles; these cells make up the cortical zones of mature follicles. Cortical cells are located external to the basement membrane which encloses the medullary compartment. Lymphoid cells are often found in breaks in the basement membrane, indicating that cell migration between cortex and medulla occurs frequently (Ackerman and Knouff, 1964). Lymphoid repopulation following X-irradiation recapitulates the normal developmental sequence of first medulla and then cortical population (unpublished observations). These findings suggest that the direction of cell traffic between the two zones is from medulla to cortex, a conclusion that is supported by autoradiographic analysis of the kinetics of bursal lymphocytes following pulse labeling with H^3-thymidine (Rubin, 1971). Finally, since the blood vessels supplying bursal follicles are located on the cortical side of the basement membrane, lymphoid cells of the medulla almost certainly would have to migrate into the cortex if they are to leave the bursa via these vessels. In conclusion, it seems likely that lymphoid cells in the cortex are immigrants from the medullary regions of bursal follicles.

Cortical and medullary cells share certain fine structural features, but differ significantly in other respects. The cytoplasm of both these cell types is richly endowed with rather evenly distributed, compact clusters of ribosomes but is poor in membranous organelles, such as rough or smooth endoplasmic reticulum (Clawson *et al.*, 1967). As a group, cells of the cortex are larger than those of the medulla. With rare exceptions, lymphoid cells of the cortex, unlike many of the medullary cells, lack detectable amounts of cytoplasmic immunoglobulins of either class (Thorbecke *et al.*, 1968; Grossi *et al.*, 1968). Finally, cortical lymphocytes divide more frequently than lymphocytes in the medulla except perhaps for those located at the most centrifugal areas of the medulla (Rubin, 1971). In other words, the cells more centrally located in the medulla appear to have a relatively long generation time and contain detectable amounts of immunoglobulins in their cytoplasms (Fig. 2), whereas the reverse is true for the more peripherally located cells of bursal follicles.

What are the fate and function of immunoglobulins synthesized by medullary cells of the bursa? Several bits of evidence suggest that these proteins are synthesized in small amounts and poorly secreted. Cytoplasmic fluorescence in medullary cells of the bursa is weak and easily quenched relative to that of mature plasma cells. This observation correlates with the fact that these cells contain abundant ribosomes, but little rough or smooth endoplasmic reticulum characteristic of cells engaged in protein secretion.

Results of a recent analysis of membrane-bound immunoglobulin on chicken lymphocytes suggest an answer to this question. In contrast to the almost complete restriction of cells containing detectable amounts of intracellular immunoglobulins to medullary areas, practically all of the lymphoid cells in the bursa carry detectable surface immunoglobulins (Kincade *et al.*, 1971). For example, an average of 70% of bursal lymphocytes from 1-day-old chicks have surface IgM determinants; around 30% bear surface IgG determinants. In normal birds, peripheral lymphocytes also carry detectable cell membrane-bound immunoglobulins of one or the other class; experimental birds lacking the bursa-dependent population of cells do not have lymphocytes which bear surface-bound immunoglobulins detectable by the same fluorescent techniques.

A reasonable and simple explanation of these observations is that the original immunoglobulins made by medullary cells are subsequently incorporated into the membranes of daughter bursal lymphocytes, where they may function as "recognition antibodies." In concordance with this view, em-

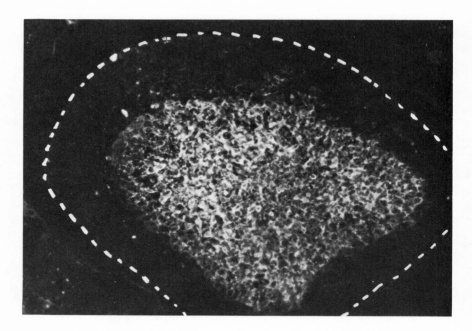

Figure 2. Pattern of immunoglobulin deposition in a mature bursal follicle as detected by fluorescein-tagged antibodies to IgM. The pattern with anti-IgG (not shown) is the same. The dotted white line outlines the outer border of the cortex. Note the virtual absence of cytoplasmic immunoglobulins in cells of the cortex, whereas the reverse is true for cells in the medulla.

bryonic bursal cells have recently been shown to have antigen-binding capability well before cells with this ability appear elsewhere (Dwyer and Warner, 1971). Further, antigen binding is inhibited significantly by pretreatment of bursal cells with antibodies to chicken immunoglobulins.

If surface immunoglobulins on bursa-derived lymphocytes are made by their ancestors in the medullary areas of bursal follicles, one might predict that the amount and extent of distribution of surface immunoglobulins would be reduced by cell division. In fact, the distribution of surface immunoglobulins on bursal lymphocytes differs from that usually observed on lymphoid cells of other tissues. Immunoglobulin "spots" tend to be spread over the entire cell membrane of bursal lymphocytes, whereas in spleen or peripheral blood cells they are more likely to occur on a circumscribed patch of the cell membrane (Kincade et al., 1971). Even if this reasoning is correct, the possibility that bursa-derived cells in the periphery are capable of synthesizing more membrane-bound immunoglobulins is not excluded. Indeed, it is attractive to think that such a mechanism may be responsible for the antigen-in-fluenced development of memory cells in peripheral tissues. Nevertheless, the "recognition antibodies" available on virgin (untouched by antigen) bursa-derived lymphocytes could be made entirely by ancestral residents of the bursal medulla.

THEORETICAL IMPLICATIONS OF GENERATION OF ANTIBODY DIVERSITY WITHIN THE BURSA

Using this background of observations and interpretations, we have con-structed a theoretical model primarily for use in designing future experiments (Fig. 3). While others have proposed a "switchover" of IgM-producing cells to become IgG-producing cells in the microevolution of specific antibody re-sponses (Nossal *et al.*, 1964; Sterzl, 1967), this model shows the switch to be a natural developmental event occurring in the induction site for plasma cell differentiation and one that is not regulated by exogenous antigens. The switch must involve repression of one part of the genome involved in immuno-globulin synthesis (constant-region gene for IgM, $C\mu$) and derepression of another (constant-region gene for IgG, $C\gamma$); just how this is controlled within the bursa is unknown.

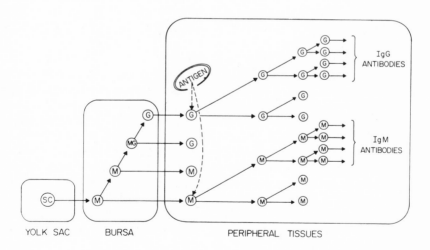

Figure 3. Hypothetical model of plasma cell differentiation in chickens. M and G refer either to cytoplasmic immunoglobulins or to the genetic capabilities for synthesis in response to antigens. This diagram does not integrate information on surface immunoglobulins of lymphoid cells along this pathway of differen-tiation.

Some of the features of this model, its relevance to plasma cell differentiation in mammals, and its possible clinical implications have been discussed elsewhere (Kincade *et al.*, 1970; Cooper *et al.*, 1971*a,b*). We will now attempt to integrate our view of plasma cell differentiation in chickens with some current theories on the generation of antibody diversity. The model proposes that major generation of antibody diversity occurs either within the bursa or prior to this point in differentiation and that little, if any, further diversification occurs in peripheral lymphoid tissues. Results of experiments reviewed earlier show that class heterogeneity is generated within the bursa and that, having left the bursa, lymphocytes are committed to synthesis of a single class of antibodies. For reasons discussed, we assume that immunoglobulins synthesized by lymphoid cells in the bursal medulla are subsequently incorporated into cell membranes, where they function as recognition antibodies. Implicit in this assumption is the concept that antigen specificity is encoded in cells of the plasma cell line during residence in the bursa.

The major theories for generation of antibody diversity have been reviewed elsewhere (*Cold Spring Harbor Symp. Quant. Biol.,* 1967; Edelman and Gall, 1969; Hood and Talmage, 1970). Simply stated, germ line theories hold that a multiplicity of variable (V) region genes have arisen through gene duplication, point mutation, and recombination during evolution, and that all of these are present in the germ line. Somatic theories begin with a number of V-region germ line genes no larger than is necessary to account for the classes and subclasses defined by sequence data. The full range of specificities is then generated by a series of mutations or recombinational events, followed by selection of useful mutants.

In the context of a germ line theory, at least two mechanisms for generation of diversity within the bursa can be proposed. The simplest is that each stem cell, on induction to begin synthesis of IgM, randomly selects from the total V-gene pool and expresses a given pair of V-region genes (V_H and V_L). The progeny of this cell will constitute a clone, defined by expression of this particular set of V genes. After a number of generations, some members of this clone undergo a switch from expression of $C\mu$ to $C\gamma$ without alteration in the expression of V genes. An alternative hypothesis is based on the premise that the genetic mechanism responsible for repression of $C\mu$ and derepression of $C\gamma$, as occurs in the switch from IgM to IgG synthesis, may act on V genes as well. In this modification of the germ line theory, a single stem cell could give rise to several clones as different V genes are sequentially expressed in its progeny.

The first mechanism, or simple germ line theory, would require that the number of stem cells entering this pathway be considerably larger than the number of V genes in the germ line. The number of different antibody specificities required by the organism to ensure recognition of any antigen is probably between 10^4 to 10^8. The lower estimate could be generated by all possible combinations of 100 V_L and 100 V_H genes. To provide a 95% probability of each of the 10^4 possible specificities being generated by random activation of a pair of V genes, 12×10^4 stem cells would be required. This number rises exponentially with an increase in the estimated number of total antibody specificities. For example, 17×10^6 stem cells would be required to express all possible combinations of 500 V_H and 500 V_L genes. For 10^4 V genes of each type (Hood and Talmage, 1970), the number of stem cells required would be astronomical.

The second mechanism, which allows for sequential activation of different germ line V genes in the progeny of a single cell, would considerably reduce the number of stem cells required. We have cited evidence that the mean generation time of bursal lymphocytes is approximately 8 hr in 15-day embryos. From this information it can be estimated that a stem cell may give rise to approximately 20 generations, comprising 10^6 progeny, during the 7 days from initial activation of IgM synthesis (14-day embryo) to the first appearance of IgG synthesis. If a probability of 10^{-2} is arbitrarily assigned for the frequency with which each division results in daughter cells expressing a different V_H or V_L gene, a single stem cell could give rise to as many as 5000 specificity clones during this period.

The economy in required numbers of stem cells achieved by the latter mechanism would be balanced by the introduction of some degeneracy in the immune response. This argument hinges on the assumption that immunoglobulin synthesized by bursal lymphocytes becomes incorporated into cell membranes and serves as recognition antibody. During cell division, each daughter cell would receive a portion of these membrane-bound antibodies. If one of the daughter cells then expresses a different V gene, it follows that this cell might be triggered by one antigen, recognized by its membrane antibody, but synthesize antibody of an entirely unrelated specificity. The proportion of cells manifesting this kind of dual specificity would vary directly with the frequency of change in the expression of a V gene. Within a few divisions, perhaps three or four, the original recognition antibody would be replaced by antibody of the new specificity. A "switch" frequency of much less than 10^{-2} would therefore result in a very small proportion of cells having dual specificities. The possibility of occurrence of cells having dual specificity is of interest because it could provide a possible explanation for situations in which only a small proportion of the immunoglobulins synthesized in response to immunization have specificity for the immunizing antigen. Moreover, the same considerations hold for theories of somatic diversification based upon a mechanism for hypermutation.

Diversification of antibody specificities by means of somatic mutations or recombination requires either a rapidly dividing cell population or special mechanisms for increasing the frequency of mutational events. A secondary, but perhaps equally important, requirement is that proliferation and mutations should not depend upon chance exposure to exogenous antigens; the rationale for this requirement is implicit in the clonal selection hypothesis (Burnet, 1957). It seems clear from the evidence cited in this review that lymphopoiesis within the bursa could meet these criteria. For example, we have estimated that a single stem cell may give rise to approximately 10^6 progeny in the time interval between the appearance of IgM-containing cells and the *initial* switch in some of the progeny to begin IgG synthesis. Further, the timing of the events of differentiation in the bursa—specifically, the initial appearance of IgM and the subsequent switch to IgG synthesis—is not influenced by exogenous antigenic stimulation. It is reasonable to assume that the rate of proliferation of bursal lymphocytes is also independent of foreign antigens. In contrast, proliferation of immunoglobulin-containing cells in peripheral lymphoid tissues is clearly antigen-dependent. According to this simple reasoning, the bursa is uniquely suited for somatic diversification.

The assumption that the first immunoglobulin synthesized by a bursal lymphocyte is eventually incorporated into the cell surface implies that any subsequent alteration in specificity will produce cells recognizing one antigen but synthesizing antibody to another. While holding for any somatic theory, this prediction becomes important only if the frequency of mutation is higher than about 10^{-2}, for reasons elaborated above. It should be emphasized that the occurrence of cells expressing one specificity in their membrane and a second in the genome is not unique to our model. Diversification by any mechanism in the progeny of an antigen-sensitive cell could produce the same result.

The assumption that the first immunoglobulin synthesized by a bursal lymphocyte is subsequently incorporated into the cell surface coupled with the observed "switchover" from IgM to IgG synthesis in the bursa also implies that cells will be found which bear surface IgM recognition antibodies but synthesize IgG antibodies in response to antigen stimulation. Indeed, cells with surface IgM and cytoplasmic IgG have been observed in rabbits (Pernis *et al.*, 1971). Although this observation seems to support the idea of an intraclonal switch from IgM to IgG synthesis as proposed in our model, it is, of course, compatible with models proposing a similar switch directed by antigens in peripheral lymphoid tissues.

CONCLUSIONS

The hypothesis that antibody diversity arises in the bursa seems compatible with either a germ line theory or a somatic theory. It therefore becomes pertinent to ask: (1) what advantages might accrue to the animal by having antibody diversity generated within a specific environment such as the bursa, and (2) what help can this model for plasma cell differentiation provide in elucidation of the mechanisms responsible for antibody diversification?

The advantages of this model arise from two characteristics of bursal lymphopoiesis: the high rate of proliferation and the apparent independence of exogenous antigenic stimulation. Together, these characteristics could allow rapid development of a full range of antibody specificities. These specificities would be available to meet the onslaught of the external environment on the neonatal animal, and would not depend on the environment for their development. The existence in the bursa of a mechanism controlling the switch from IgM to IgG synthesis provides another advantage. All of the different specificities which are generated during IgM synthesis will be associated, after the switch, with IgG as well. According to the simple germ line theory, the specificity of a given clone is set at the time of initial activation for IgM synthesis. Thus each and every clone, defined by expression of a given set of V genes, would be represented by cells synthesizing IgM and others synthesizing IgG. The other two mechanisms mentioned above allow alterations in specificity genes, either by mutations or by expression of a different V-region gene, after initial activation. Either mechanism could permit development of new specificity clones after the switch to IgG synthesis; these might not be represented by IgM-producing cells. However, the full complement of specificities developed before the switch would be associated with both IgM and IgG antibodies. Therefore, this model ensures that most antibody specificities will have the specific biological advantages conferred by association with each heavy-chain class.

If this model for plasma cell differentiation proves useful in elucidating the mechanisms responsible for generation of antibody diversity, it will do so by defining the time and place in which these mechanisms are operable. For example, several proposed mechanisms for generating somatic diversity involve specific enzymes which cleave and repair V-gene DNA (Brenner and Milstein, 1966) or which catalyze intrachromasomal recombination and specific insertion of episomal DNA (Gally and Edelman, 1970). Our model suggests a time and a specific organ where evidence for such enzymatic mechanisms might be sought. Similarly, mechanisms responsible for derepression of genes controlling immunoglobulin synthesis, and for the switch from IgM to IgG synthesis, should be approachable in this site. We submit that lymphoid differentiation within the bursa, involving a series of genetic events leading to the expression of analyzable end products in a relatively uniform cell population, offers unique opportunities to probe both the molecular basis of differentiation in general and the mechanisms for generation of antibody diversity. Finally, if this model has relevance to plasma cell differentiation in mammals, as we believe to be the case, the search for a mammalian bursa equivalent becomes even more important.

REFERENCES

Ackerman, G. A., and Knouff, R. A., 1964. Lymphocytopoietic activity in the bursa of Fabricius. In Good, R. A., and Gabrielsen, A. E., eds., *The Thymus in Immunobiology*, Hoeber-Harper, New York, pp. 123-149.

Bockman, D. E., and Cooper, M. D., 1971. Fine structural analysis of pinocytosis in lymphoid follicle-associated epithelium in chick bursa and rabbit appendix. *Fed. Proc.* 30:511, abst.

Brenner, S., and Milstein, C., 1966. Origin of antibody variation. *Nature* 211:242.

Burnet, F. M., 1957. A modification of Jerne's theory of antibody production using the concept of clonal selection. *Aust. J. Sci.* 20:67.

Clawson, C. C., Cooper, M. D., and Good, R. A., 1967. Lymphocyte fine structure in the bursa of Fabricius, the thymus, and the germinal centers. *Lab. Invest.* 16:407.

Cold Spring Harbor Symposia on Quantitative Biology, 1967. Vol. 32: *Antibodies*, Cold Spring Harbor Laboratory of Quantitative Biology, Cold Spring Harbor, L.I., New York.

Cooper, M. D., Peterson, R. D. A., South, M. A., and Good, R. A., 1966a. The functions of the thymus system and the bursa system in the chicken. *J. Exptl. Med.* 123:75.

Cooper, M. D., Schwartz, M. M., and Good, R. A., 1966b. Restoration of gamma globulin production in agammaglobulinemic chickens. *Science* 151:471.

Cooper, M. D., Cain, W. A., Van Alten, P. J., and Good, R. A., 1969. Development and function of the immunoglobulin-producing system: I. Effect of bursectomy at different stages of development on germinal centers, plasma cells, immunoglobulins and antibody production. *Internat. Arch. Allergy* 35:242.

Cooper, M. D., Kincade, P. W., and Lawton, A. R., 1971a. Thymus and bursal function in immunologic development: A new theoretical model of plasma cell differentiation. In Kagan, B. M., and Stiehm, E. R., eds., *Immunologic Incompetence,* Year Book Medical Publishers, Chicago, pp. 81-101.

Cooper, M. D., Kincade, P. W., Bockman, D. E., and Lawton, A. R., 1971b. A new theoretical model of plasma cell differentiation. In Lindahl-Kiessling et al., eds., *Morphological and Functional Aspects of Immunity,* Plenum Publishing Corp., New York, pp. 17-24.

Durkin, H. G., Theis, G. A., and Thorbecke, G. J., 1971. Homing of cells from the bursa of Fabricius to germinal centers in the chicken spleen. In Lindahl-Kiessling et al., eds., *Morphological and Functional Aspects of Immunity,* Plenum Publishing Corp., New York, pp. 119-128.

Dwyer, J. M., and Warner, N. L., 1971. Antigen binding cells in embryonic chicken bursa and thymus. *Nature New Biol.* 229:210.

Edelman, G. M., and Gall, W. E., 1969. The antibody problem. *Ann. Rev. Biochem.* 38:415.

Gally, J. A., and Edelman, G. M., 1970. Somatic translocation of antibody genes. *Nature* 227:341.

Grossi, C. E., Genta, V., Ferrarini, M., and Zaccheo, D., 1968. Localization of immunoglobulins in the developing chicken bursa of Fabricius. *Rev. Franc. Etud. Clin. Biol.* 5:497.

Hood, L., and Talmage, D. W., 1970. Mechanism of antibody diversity: Germ line basis for variability. *Science* 168:325.

Kincade, P. W., and Cooper, M. D., 1971. Development and distribution of immunoglobulin-containing cells in the chicken: An immunofluorescent analysis using purified antibodies to μ, γ and light chains. *J. Immunol.* 106:371.

Kincade, P. W., Lawton, A. R., Bockman, D. E., and Cooper, M. D., 1970. Suppression of immunoglobulin G synthesis as a result of antibody-mediated suppression of immunoglobulin M synthesis in chickens. *Proc. Natl. Acad. Sci.* 67:1918.

Kincade, P. W., Lawton, A. R., and Cooper, M. D., 1971. Restriction of surface immunoglobulin determinants to lymphocytes of the plasma cell line. *J. Immunol.* 106:1421.

Moore, M. A. S., and Owen, J. J. T., 1966. Experimental studies on the development of the bursa of Fabricius. *Develop. Biol.* 14:40.

Nossal, G. J. V., Szenberg, A., Ada, G. L., and Austin, G. M., 1964. Single cell studies on 19S antibody production. *J. Exptl. Med.* 119:485.

Pernis, B., Forni, L., and Amante, L., 1971. Immunoglobulins as cell receptors. Conference on immunoglobulins. *New York Acad. Sci.,* in press.

Rubin, Eva, 1971. The kinetics of cellular proliferation in the bursa of Fabricius. Master's thesis, University of Alabama in Birmingham, manuscript in preparation.

Sterzl, J., 1967. Factors determining the differentiation pathways of immunocompetent cells. *Cold Spring Harbor Symp. Quant. Biol.* 32:493.

Thompson, J. H., and Cooper, M. D., 1971. Functional deficiency of autologous implants of the bursa of Fabricius in chickens. *Transplantation* 11:71.

Thorbecke, G. J., Warner, N. L., Hochwald, G. M., and Ohanian, S. H., 1968. Immune globulin production by the bursa of Fabricius of young chickens. *Immunology* 15:123.

Van Meter, R., Good, R. A., and Cooper, M. D., 1969. Ontogeny of circulating immunoglobulins in normal, bursectomized and irradiated chickens. *J. Immunol.* 102:370.

Warner, N. L., Uhr, J. W., Thorbecke, G. J., and Ovary, Z., 1969. Immunoglobulins, antibodies and the bursa of Fabricius: Induction of agammaglobulinemia and the loss of all antibody-forming capacity by hormonal bursectomy. *J. Immunol.* 103:1317.

Chapter 3

The Mammalian "Bursa Equivalent": Does Lymphoid Differentiation Along Plasma Cell Lines Begin in the Gut-Associated Lymphoepithelial Tissues (GALT) of Mammals?

Max D. Cooper* and Alexander R. Lawton†

Spain Research Laboratories
Departments of Pediatrics and Microbiology
University of Alabama Medical Center
Birmingham, Alabama

INTRODUCTION

Definition of the induction sites for development of the antibody-producing line of cells in mammals seems to us one of the most important problems in contemporary immunobiology. With the discovery in the early 1960s of the role of the mammalian thymus in the development of immuno-competent cells (Good and Gabrielsen, 1964), it was tempting to assume that the thymus was also central to development of antibody-producing cells. This idea was particularly attractive since deficient antibody responsiveness was frequently found in animals subjected to removal of the thymus early in life. Information gained since refuted this possibility and directed attention away from the thymus in the search for the sites of origin of the plasma cell line.

In 1963, Archer *et al.*, observed that, unlike lymphoid development in lymph nodes and spleen, lymphopoiesis in the appendix occurred normally in

Supported by grants from the National Institutes of Health (AI-08345 and RR-05349) and The American Cancer Society.

* American Cancer Society Faculty Research Associate, Professor of Pediatrics, and Associate Professor of Microbiology.

† U.S.P.H.S. Special Postdoctoral Fellow (AI-42973).

rabbits deprived of their thymuses at birth (Archer *et al.*, 1963, 1964). Further, they demonstrated that removal of the appendix in newborn rabbits impaired development of antibody responsiveness and enhanced the antibody deficiency and lymphopenia produced by neonatal thymectomy (Sutherland *et al.*, 1964). Finally, these investigators noted striking morphological similarities between the rabbit appendix and the chicken bursa of Fabricius, an organ known to be necessary for normal development of humoral immunity in this animal (Glick *et al.*, 1956). They concluded that the rabbit appendix was a central lymphoid organ, like the thymus and the bursa. They suggested that other gut-associated lymphoepithelial tissues in the rabbit might also serve in such a capacity.

In 1962, Warner *et al.* and later others (Aspinall *et al.*, 1963; Janković and Isvaneski, 1963) provided evidence which indicated that in chickens the thymus and the bursa of Fabricius exert different influences on immunological development. This concept was confirmed in a series of experiments which defined two separate lines of lymphoid differentiation in this animal (Cooper *et al.*, 1965, 1966*a*; Clawson *et al.*, 1967): (a) a thymus-dependent line responsible for cellular immunity, and (b) an additional avenue of lymphoid differentiation directed along plasma cell lines which begins its development in the bursa and is responsible for humoral immunity. In these experiments it was shown that immunological deficits and biological consequences in chickens with severely impaired thymus-system development were the same as those which followed thymectomy in newborn mice. These results, taken together with observations in humans with various immunological deficiency diseases (Peterson *et al.*, 1965; DiGeorge, 1965), indicated that the thymus serves the same role in development of the immune system in birds as it does in mammals; the observations also indicated that the thymus is not the source of antibody-producing cells in either man or chickens, a conclusion that was quickly confirmed in mice (Davies *et al.*, 1967; Tyan and Herzenberg, 1968; Mitchell and Miller, 1968).

It was postulated, therefore, that mammals should also have a separate site for induction of plasma cell differentiation, a mammalian homologue of the avian bursa of Fabricius (Cooper *et al.*, 1966*a*). It was further proposed that gut-associated lymphoepithelial tissues (GALT), such as Peyer's patch type of tissues, might fulfill this role along with the appendix in those mammals which have this lymphoid appendage. Initial support for this theory was soon provided by experiments which showed that removal of GALT plus near lethal whole-body irradiation in young adult rabbits resulted in persistent impairment of humoral immunity but had no long-term effects on the thymus system of lymphocytes and cellular immunity (Cooper *et al.*, 1966*c*).

The GALT hypothesis, simply stated, proposed that stem cells of hematopoietic tissue origin migrate to special microenvironments in close association with intestinal epithelium where they are influenced to begin lymphoid differentiation. The lymphoid follicles in these locations in turn supply the rest of the body with a specialized population of lymphoid cells capable of populating germinal centers, becoming plasma cells, and producing immunoglobulins. This hypothesis was proposed as a model amenable to experimental dissection, using as a guide the knowledge gained and to be gained from study of the easily manipulated bursal system in chickens. Since this theory was conceived, a considerable amount of experimental data has accumulated relating to mammalian GALT. It is the purpose of this review to relate this information to predictions originally made by or subsequently incorporated into the GALT theory of plasma cell differentiation in an attempt to find if the data support or refute the theory. We will also attempt to draw attention to certain areas where further information is needed.

PREDICTIONS IN THE GALT THEORY

1. *Lymphopoiesis occurring in organized lymphoid follicles of GALT should be developmentally independent of the thymus.*

Attention was focused on the rabbit appendix as a central lymphoid tissue with the discovery that follicular lymphopoiesis occurring there was thymus-independent (Archer *et al.*, 1964; Sutherland *et al.*, 1964, 1970). Follicular lymphoid development has also been observed in the Peyer's patches and appendix of humans with agenesis or congenital lymphoid aplasia of the thymus (Matsaniotis *et al.*, 1966; DiGeorge, 1968). Similarly, development of lymphoid follicles is not impaired in Peyer's patches of congenitally athymic mice (DeSousa, 1969). This evidence clearly affirms the thymus independence of follicular lymphopoiesis in GALT of several species of mammals. Since germinal center formation in other sites shares this characteristic, this information does not provide evidence on the central nature of these lymphopoietic sites nor does it provide information regarding the stage in differentiation of their constituent lymphoid cells.

Two additional characteristics of GALT in mammals might be emphasized here since we believe they are likely sources for interpretive errors in evaluating results of experiments relating to GALT. The first is that some thymus-derived cells migrate to the mammalian GALT (Gowans and Knight, 1964; Evans *et al.*, 1967; Davies, 1969; Raff and Owen, 1971). Characteristically, they occur in areas outside of the organized lymphoid follicles (Sutherland *et al.*, 1970; DeSousa *et al.*, 1969). By their location alone, GALT are particularly vulnerable to invasion by foreign materials. Furthermore, the epithelium overlying GALT seems to be especially prone to penetration by elements from the intestinal lumen (Friedenstein and Goncharenko, 1965;

Shimizu and Andrew, 1967; Hanaoka et al., 1971; Bockman and Cooper, 1971). Therefore, it might be expected that immunocompetent thymus-derived lymphocytes would often be attracted to these locations. This may account for the observation that in the mouse some thymus and lymph node cells eventually make their way to Peyer's patches and are transient residents there during recovery from total-body X-irradiation (Evans et al., 1967). It could also explain why thoracic duct lymphocytes traffic to Peyer's patches in rats (Gowans and Knight, 1964) as well as the fact that cells are found in the human and rabbit appendix which respond to phytohemagglutinin stimulation (Astaldi et al., 1968; Daguillard and Richter, 1970), a property characteristic of thymus-dependent lymphocytes. With the possible exception of very young mice, however, the Peyer's patches in the mouse contain the smallest percentage of thymus-derived cells seen in any organized lymphoid tissue of the body (Davies, 1969; Raff and Owen, 1971). Thus we would suggest that thymus-derived cells appear in GALT in response to antigenic invasion. This does not constitute convincing evidence against the idea that GALT are the sites of lymphoid differentiation along plasma cell lines. Such an argument is comparable to the use of plasma cell occurrence in the thymus as evidence against that organ's primary role in lymphopoiesis.

Another feature of GALT that seems worthy of mention is the apparent sensitivity of GALT lymphopoiesis, like bursal and thymic lymphopoiesis, to the involutional effects of stress which may be mediated by corticosteroids. Misleading impressions can be gained when this fact is not taken into consideration. For example, gross inspection of the intestines of athymic humans following death after prolonged and stressful illness originally suggested that Peyer's patches did not develop normally in athymic individuals. However, normal GALT development has since been observed in athymic infants who died suddenly without long stressful illness, suggesting that stress and not the absence of thymus tissue was the critical factor in the former cases (DiGeorge, 1968).

2. *Stem cells of hemopoietic tissue origin should migrate to GALT, where they are influenced to begin differentiation along plasma cell lines.*

We believe that solid evidence in favor of or against this requirement must be obtained in order to prove or refute conclusively the GALT hypothesis. However, we know of no currently available evidence which incisively deals with this question. One experimental approach to this issue which seemed reasonably simple was to select an animal in which all of the GALT could be removed, heavily irradiate that animal, supply it with embryonic stem cells, and then evaluate its humoral immunity. Such experiments have been performed in the rabbit, and the results are unambiguous (Perey et al., 1968, 1970). In those animals subjected to GALT removal, primary antibody responses to antigens given immediately before lethal whole-body irradiation were severely stunted or abolished. Control animals subjected to sham surgery, immunized just prior to lethal whole-body X-ray exposure, and then given fetal liver cells were capable of brisk primary antibody responses. These results were thought to provide evidence that donor stem cells of fetal liver origin were induced to become antibody producers under the influence of the recipient's GALT. Recent observations have made us doubt this interpretation. When young rabbits homozygous for one immunoglobulin allotype were heavily irradiated and given fetal liver cells from rabbits homozygous for another immunoglobulin allotype, only recipient immunoglobulins were produced for several weeks; cells producing immunoglobulins of the donor allotype did not appear until more than 2 months had elapsed (Lawton et al., manuscript in preparation). Therefore, a more reasonable interpretation of the results obtained in the experiments cited above is that cells with antibody-producing potential in rabbit GALT can survive heavy exposure to X-rays. Observations in mice subjected to lethal whole-body irradiation and saved with injections of bone marrow and lymphocytes are interesting in this regard; most of the dividing cells in Peyer's patches are host cells during the first 3 weeks after irradiation (Evans et al., 1967). Eventually, however, Peyer's patches in such mice are repopulated by bone marrow cells of donor origin.

In our view, the most critical test of the GALT hypothesis is to determine whether fetal stem cells can be influenced to begin synthesis of immunoglobulins in an animal entirely lacking Peyer's patches and appendix. The positive counterpart of this experiment would be to show whether or not GALT locations are the first where fetal stem cells gain the capability of producing immunoglobulins. Although either of these approaches is likely to be difficult, both seem to be experimentally feasible.

3. *Development of organized lymphoid follicles in GALT should (a) occur before follicular development occurs in non-thymus dependent areas of peripheral lymphoid tissue, (b) begin before immunoglobulin-producing cells exist elsewhere in the body, and (c) not depend on exogenous antigenic stimulation.*

The reasons for these requirements are implicit in the GALT hypothesis and are based on the observations that thymic and avian bursal lymphopoiesis are vigorous in relatively antigen-sheltered environments such as exist during embryonic life and under germ-free conditions.

It has been reported that in sheep (Silverstein and Prendergast, 1971), bovine (Schultz et al., 1970), and human embryos (Matsumura et al., 1968; Gitlin, 1971), lymphoid development in the intestines significantly lags behind the development of antibody-producing cells in peripheral lymphoid tissues. We have used the fetal pig as a model to investigate this problem (Chapman et al., submitted for publication), since this animal is sheltered by a six-layered placenta which is impervious to most antigens, including maternal immunoglobulins. We were unable to locate lymphoid follicles along the intestine of pig embryos until several weeks beyond the age at which immunoglobulin-containing cells could be found easily by immunofluorescence techniques. Before embracing the obvious conclusion that antibody-producing cells in peripheral lymphoid tissues could not have come from GALT, we examined serial longitudinal sections of the entire intestines of very young pig embryos. Peyer's patch lymphoid development could be found in 11 cm pig embryos (estimated gestational age of 50 days), whereas IgM-containing cells were first found in peripheral lymphoid tissues of 12.5 or 13 cm embryos; development of primary and secondary lymphoid follicles in non-thymus dependent areas of spleen and mesenteric lymph nodes was a later event. The lymphoid follicles in Peyer's patches of embryos showed a progressive increase in size with advancing age. These observations indicate that lymphoid development of Peyer's patches does not require exposure to food or intestinal microflora. They show this type of lymphoid development to be as independent of stimulation by exogenous antigens as lymphopoiesis in the thymus. Our studies also demonstrate the kind of careful scrutiny needed to find the earliest stages of Peyer's patch development.

Lymphoid follicles have been demonstrated in rabbit GALT during embryonic life (Crabb and Kelsall, 1940), whereas immunoglobulin-containing cells cannot be found in peripheral lymphoid tissues until after birth (Adler *et al.*, 1967). Small Peyer's patches have been observed in a human embryo at approximately 11 weeks of gestational age, and well-developed lymphoid follicles can be found in the appendix of humans by 16 weeks of embryonic life (unpublished observations). It is also well known that follicular lymphoid development occurs in Peyer's patches of germ-free mice. It has been stated that corticomedullary organization of these follicles only occurs in germ-free mice given antigens by mouth (Pollard and Sharon, 1970); we have been unable to confirm this observation. However, corticomedullary organization of the lymphoid follicles in both mammalian GALT and the avian bursa is a postembryonic development and may depend upon antigen exposure.

4. *GALT should be the first sites of development of cells with the ability to produce immunoglobulins.*

If GALT are the induction sites for lymphoid development in mammals, it is reasonable to expect that immunoglobulin-producing cells should occur first in these locations, as is the case for the bursa of Fabricius in birds. Presently, there is little available evidence on this critical point. By use of a fairly sensitive technique of detection of immunoglobulin synthesis, the rabbit appendix was found to be an early site of immunoglobulin production (Thorbecke, 1960). Immunofluorescence should be an even more sensitive technique for analysis of this question. Using this technique, we have been unable to detect immunoglobulin-containing cells in the earliest follicles developing along the intestines of pigs and rabbits. The difficulty in locating the earliest Peyer's patches has prevented optimum fixation of the tissues, however, and the relatively high background fluorescence in our studies has prevented detection of cells with relatively small amounts of cytoplasmic immunoglobulins. It is also reasonable to expect that the first lymphocytes with membrane-bound immunoglobulins should occur in the mammalian equivalent of the bursa of Fabricius. Since the search for these cells should present less technical difficulty, our current efforts are in this direction.

5. *Early removal of GALT should impair development of humoral immunity but should not affect cellular immunity.*

The GALT hypothesis specifically states that the rest of the body receives lymphoid cells with antibody-producing capabilities from the organized lymphoid follicles of GALT. Therefore, early removal of GALT, like early removal of the bursa, should result in a selective deficiency of that line of cells having the capacity for immunoglobulin production. In fact, removal of GALT before onset of cellular traffic from this site should result in agammaglobulinemia. Unfortunately, this is more easily said than done. In most mammalian species, GALT are extensively distributed along the small intestines and they are richly endowed with lymphopoietic activity long before birth. The rabbit has been the most suitable model for studies involving extirpation of GALT because in this animal GALT development is not extensive at birth (Crabb and Kelsall, 1940; Ackerman, 1966; Stramignoni and Mollo, 1968) and involves only approximately eight intestinal patches besides the easily removable appendix. Indeed, when fully developed, the appendix alone probably represents more than half of the rabbit GALT since it is relatively enormous in size and loaded with organized follicles.

Since the original studies by Archer *et al.* (1963, 1964) and Sutherland *et al.* (1964), many investigators have shown that early appendectomy, with or without whole-body X-irradiation, impairs humoral immunity in rabbits (Konda *et al.*, 1966, 1967; Hanaoka *et al.*, 1967; Cooper *et al.*, 1968; Perey *et al.*, 1968b; Perey and Good, 1968a). Removal of all GALT is much more difficult, and, to date, removal of the Peyer's patches has not been possible in rabbits much younger than 2 weeks of age. Since Peyer's patches of rabbits may contain many lymphoid follicles at birth, there is considerable opportunity for lymphoid cells of Peyer's patches to migrate elsewhere over the first weeks of life. Nevertheless, it has been possible to show selective impairment of humoral immunity in rabbits subjected to early removal of GALT, whereas animals subjected to appropriate control surgery of the intestine showed no immunological impairment (Cooper *et al.*, 1968; Perey *et al.*, 1968b). The animals subjected to GALT extirpation were relatively lymphopenic, deficient in germinal centers, hypogammaglobulinemic, poor antibody producers, highly susceptible to "autoimmune" phenomena, and unable to survive epidemic diarrhea. On the other hand, these same animals were able to reject skin allografts and express delayed allergy as well as normal rabbits. As mentioned earlier, similar results have been obtained in older rabbits subjected to removal of their GALT and then exposed to lethal or near lethal whole-body X-irradiation (Cooper et al., 1966c).

It is clear that early removal of a large part or nearly all of the rabbit GALT selectively impairs development of the immunoglobulin-producing line of cells; the effects are similar to those observed in chickens subjected to bursectomy in the first few weeks of life (Chang et al., 1957). In both of these instances, development of humoral immunity was significantly advanced before removal of the GALT. It is not surprising, therefore, that development of humoral immunity was only stunted, not abolished. Nevertheless, the results are compatible with the hypothesis that mammalian GALT supply the rest of the body with lymphoid cells of the plasma cell line.

Alternatively, it has been suggested that the immunological effects of GALT removal are simply due to the huge mass of lymphoid tissue removed by appendectomy, with or without excision of Peyer's patches. This possibility seems unlikely since many of these studies employed appendectomy of newborn rabbits and very little lymphoid development can be found in the appendix of the newborn rabbit (Crabb and Kelsall, 1940; Ackerman, 1966; Stramignoni and Mollo, 1968).

It has been reported that intrauterine removal of the entire intestine of sheep embryos does not prevent development of germinal centers, plasma cells, and antibody production (Silverstein and Prendergast, 1971). In these experiments, the intestines were removed at least 2 weeks beyond the age at which sheep embryos can already mount vigorous antibody responses to certain antigens. Therefore, the results might best be compared with the effects of relatively late removal of the bursa in chickens. Even so, using sufficient numbers of sheep embryos and quantitative assessment of humoral immunity, this model could provide useful information on the role of the GALT in this species. It is of some interest that the same investigators found that thymectomy of very young sheep embryos failed to alter development of cellular immunity.

6. *Lymphoid cells of GALT follicles should (a) be capable of selectively populating thymus-independent areas of peripheral lymphoid tissues with cells of plasma cell lineage, (b) be capable of responding to appropriate antigen exposure with antibody synthesis, and (c) be incapable of producing graft vs. host disease.*

By lead shielding of the rabbit appendix or the mouse Peyer's patch and exposure of the rest of the body to lethal or nearly lethal X-irradiation (Jacobson et al., 1950, 1961; Süssdorf, 1959, 1960; Süssdorf and Draper, 1956), it has been possible to define the capabilities of GALT cells in repopulation of lymphoid tissues throughout the body. Both the rabbit appendix and mouse Peyer's patches are capable of seeding cells to lymph nodes and spleen which have antibody-producing capabilities. Most of the early lymphoid re-population that is fostered by irradiation-protected Peyer's patches of mice appears to be directed along plasma cell lines, in contrast to the small lympho-cytes which are seeded from the irradiation-protected thymus (Miller, 1966). On the other hand, cells in the shielded Peyer's patches failed to contribute either to bone marrow regeneration or to granulocytic, megakaryocytic, or erythrocytic regeneration elsewhere. In the rabbit experiments, cells migrated from the irradiation-protected appendix to the mesenteric lymph nodes and spleen and began to produce hemolytic antibodies to sheep erythrocytes in these secondary locations. These observations were made in an elegant series of experiments (Jacobson, 1950, 1961; Süssdorf, 1959, 1961; Süssdorf and Draper, 1956) which were begun in 1950 and completed before the present-day concepts of central lymphoid tissues and of separate lines of lymphoid differentiation were formulated. Most subsequent investigations of mammalian GALT have provided results that are amazingly complementary to the infor-mation obtained in these irradiation recovery experiments. For example, the investigations which involved analysis of the effects of GALT removal on humoral immunity are the obverse of the studies outlined above; other close parallels can be noted below.

When antigens are given via the usual routes in chickens (Dent and Good, 1965; Janković and Mitrović, 1967), rabbits (Good et al., 1969; Henry et al., 1970; Faulk et al., 1970; Hanaoka and Waksman, 1970), rats (Cooper and Turner, 1969), mice (Coppola et al., 1970), and hamsters (Bienenstock and Dolezel, 1971), relatively few antibody-secreting cells are subsequently found in the GALT. Nevertheless, GALT cells are perfectly capable of developing into antibody producers when appropriate antigen exposure is provided. Following injection of an antigen directly into rat Peyer's patches, antibody-producing cells occur locally, but even then they are about tenfold fewer than in the draining mesenteric node (Cooper and Turner, 1967). Injection of a few sheep erythrocytes into a Peyer's patch results in a rapid seeding of cells secreting IgM antibodies and of memory cells to the draining mesenteric lymph node and spleen (Cooper and Turner, 1969). Cells capable of producing IgM anti-bodies can leave the shielded appendix of an irradiated rabbit within 30 min following antigen injection (Hanaoka and Waksman, 1970; Hanaoka et al., 1970). Cells from mouse Peyer's patches give rise to hemolytic plaques when stimulated with sheep erythrocytes in lethally irradiated syngeneic recipients (Brody and Hencin, 1969). Rabbit sacculus rotundus cells give rise to plaque-forming cells in irradiated recipients when given along with sheep erythrocytes (Abdou and Richter, 1970). Finally, cell cultures prepared from Peyer's patches of rabbits respond to sheep erythrocytes with antibody production comparable to that produced by spleen cells under similar conditions (Henry et al., 1970). These results clearly document that mammalian GALT, like the avian bursa (Gilmour et al., 1970); contain cells fully capable of response to antigen with antibody production and secretion but under normal conditions they produce little antibody for secretion in situ. These observations are clearly compatible with the idea that mammalian GALT are central lymphoid tissues having the same functions as the avian bursa of Fabricius.

Finally, it has been shown that cells of mouse Peyer's patches, when given to irradiated recipients, selectively repopulate the non-thymus dependent areas (including germinal centers) of the spleen and that they possess relatively little graft vs. host reactivity (Heim et al., 1970; Cooper et al., 1967). The results reinforce the suggestion that mouse Peyer's patches share more functional similarities with the chicken bursa than with the mouse thymus, lymph nodes, or spleen.

7. *Lymphoid follicles in GALT of mammals should be similar to bursal follicles of chickens in their (a) general architecture, (b) fine structural characteristics of constituent cells, (c) cellular kinetics, (d) immunoglobulin distribution, (e) antigen-handling abilities, and (f) relationship to specialized intestinal epithelium.*

The lymphoid follicles of mammalian Peyer's patches and the appendix are frequently regarded as structural analogues of the germinal centers or secondary follicles of lymph nodes and spleen, although it is difficult to find support to such an assumption. In fact, the lymphoid follicles of mammalian GALT are distinctly different from the secondary lymphoid follicles seen in lymph nodes and spleen in their general architecture, cellular kinetics, antigen relationships, and immunoglobulin distribution. On the other hand, their resemblance in these ways to the lymphoid follicles of the chicken bursa is striking.

The lymphoid follicles of GALT develop in close relationship to a very specialized epithelium which is distinct from surrounding intestinal epithelium (Shimizu and Andrew, 1967; Faulk et al., 1970). For example, the epithelium associated with lymphoid follicles of the rabbit appendix and the chicken bursa has been shown to have pinocytotic capabilities that are not shared by the epithelial cells of adjacent villi (Bockman and Cooper, 1971). This pinocytotic mechanism for sampling of intestinal contents may be necessary for lymphoid differentiation in GALT follicles since isolation of rabbit Peyer's patches and appendix (Perey and Good, 1968b; Stramignoni et al., 1969), or the chicken bursa (Thompson and Cooper, 1971), from the normal flow of intestinal contents aborts lymphoid development in these tissues.

Early in development, the lymphoid follicles of mammalian GALT are not divided into medullary and cortical zones; this kind of compartmentalization appears to be a postembryonic development in those animals which have been examined. This sequence of development parallels the development of lymphoid follicles in the chicken bursa. The similarity of the overall architecture of the lymphoid follicles of the rabbit appendix and the chicken bursa is illustrated in Fig. 1. The fine structure of the lymphoid cells in these locations is also strikingly similar in the two animals (Clawson et al., 1967; Bockman and Cooper, 1971; Faulk et al., 1970). One difference is that the cortical and medullary zones of mammalian GALT follicles are not separated by a layer of epithelial cells as is the case in avian bursal follicles. In both, the lymphoid cells of the cortex are larger and divide more rapidly than the lymphoid cells of the medullary areas of the follicles (Faulk et al., 1970; Meuwissen et al., 1969a; Rubin, 1971), whereas the reverse relationship is true for secondary follicles of lymph nodes and spleen. In addition, many of the medullary lymphoid cells have detectable amounts of immunoglobulins, as shown in Fig. 2. We have observed a similar pattern of immunoglobulin distribution in the appendix and/or Peyer's patches of humans, pigs, mice, and rabbits (unpublished observations). Immunoglobulins found in the medullary zones of individual GALT follicles include multiple immunoglobulin classes in all of the animals analyzed and more than one immunoglobulin allotype in heterozygous rabbits. By contrast, in germinal centers we find only an occasional lymphoid cell with detectable immunoglobulin of a single class and allotype, although we sometimes see surface staining for multiple immunoglobulin determinants on reticular cells of germinal centers.

GALT follicles also differ from organized lymphoid follicles of lymph nodes and spleen in that they lack antigen-trapping dendritic histiocytes which are characteristically seen in germinal centers in other locations (Faulk et al., 1970; Hanaoka and Waksman, 1970; Bienenstock and Dolezel, 1971). This observation probably provides at least a partial explanation as to why lymphoid cells of mammalian GALT and the avian bursa do not differentiate into antibody-secreting cells in situ. This is not to say that antigens have no influence on the lymphoid cells in these locations, since it is clear that foreign substances, including intestinal microorganisms, frequently penetrate the follicle-associated epithelium of GALT and thereby enter the lymphoid follicles.

CONCLUSIONS

Evidence obtained from several mammalian species indicates that, like the lymphopoiesis which occurs in the avian bursa of Fabricius, lymphopoiesis in the follicles of Peyer's patches and the appendix (a) is thymus-independent, (b) develops independently of stimulation by exogenous antigens, (c) begins before significant lymphoid development occurs in thymus-independent regions of lymph nodes and spleen, (d) develops before immunoglobulin-contain-

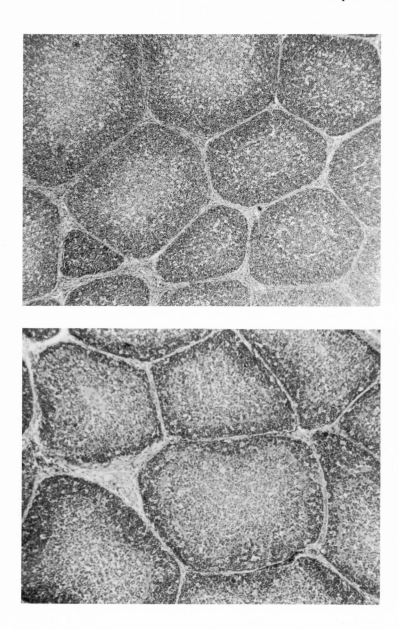

Figure 1. (a) Cross section of the lymphoid follicles in the large Peyer's patch located at the ileocecal junction of rabbits. The corticomedullary organization of these follicles is remarkably similar to (b) that in follicles of the chicken bursa of Fabricius.

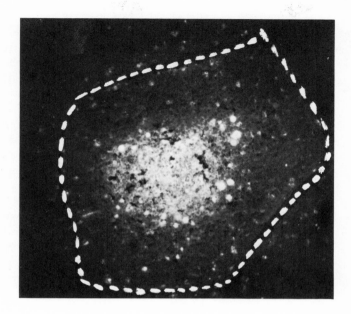

Figure 2. Pattern of immunoglobulin deposition in a lymphoid follicle of the rabbit appendix as detected by fluorescein-tagged antibodies to IgM. The patterns seen with anti-IgG and anti-IgA (not shown) are virtually the same. The dotted white line outlines the outer border of the cortex. Note the confinement of immunoglobulin deposition to cells of the medullary region. Compare with Figure 1 (this chapter) and with IgM distribution within a lymphoid follicle of the chicken bursa of Fabricius (Figure 2, Chapter 2).

ing cells appear elsewhere, (e) involves an abundance of cells with ultrastructural characteristics that are similar to those of the lymphoid cells of the avian bursa of Fabricius, (f) involves lymphoid cells with antibody-producing capabilities, (g) produces lymphoid cells capable of selective population of thymus-independent areas of peripheral lymphoid tissues with a line of cells which includes lymphoid cells of germinal centers and plasma cells, (h) is necessary for normal development of cells in thymus-independent areas of peripheral lymphoid tissues which are responsible for humoral immunity, (i) develops beneath specialized areas of intestinal epithelium, and (g) differs from secondary follicles of peripheral lymphoid tissues in general structural organization, cellular kinetics, pattern of immunoglobulin deposition, and antigen-trapping capability.

Several critical predictions of the GALT hypothesis remain untested. For example, it should be possible using techniques that are presently available to determine if during development cells with immunoglobulin-producing capabilities occur in Peyer's patches and the appendix before they can be found in other sites. If GALT are the only sites where this type of lymphoid differentiation can be induced in mammals, it should be possible to show that stem cells of yolk sac or embryonic liver origin must migrate to these locations in order to begin a plasma cell line of differentiation. Conversely, if a method can be devised which would prevent lymphoid development of GALT, agammaglobulinemia should ensue. Although it seems likely that Peyer's patches and the appendix will prove to have the same functions in all mammalian species, this also needs experimental analysis.

Although never formally stated as a theory, the concept that the bone marrow serves as the induction site for B lymphocytes in mice seems to have gained wide acceptance. It seems pertinent to briefly comment on evidence supporting this concept. The bone marrow of mature mammals is clearly the major repository of lymphoid stem cells. These cells are capable of reconstituting the lymphoid organs of lethally irradiated mice, or of humans congenitally lacking both cellular and humoral immunity (Micklem *et al.*, 1966; Meuwissen *et al.*, 1969*b*). Mouse bone marrow can also serve as an experimental source of lymphocytes which have the capacity to differentiate into antibody-secreting cells under proper conditions of antigenic stimulation and cooperation with thymic-dependent lymphocytes (Claman *et al.*, 1966; Mitchell and Miller, 1968; Davies, 1969; Miller and Mitchell, 1969). The presence of cells mediating these two functions in this site has led to use of the term "bone marrow-derived" to refer to cells involved in humoral immunity in the same manner that "thymus-derived" is used to refer to cells mediating cellular immunity. However, in order to make the bone marrow-derived concept equivalent to a bone marrow induction site theory, one would either need to assume that (a) bone marrow stem cells and bone marrow B lymphocytes are the same, or (b) bone marrow stem cells can be converted *in situ* into B lymphocytes.

We assume for this argument that the stem cell is uncommitted and that commitment to recognition of a given antigen comprises a later stage of differentiation. This assumption is apparently valid for the thymus system (Stutman and Good, 1971); proof that it holds for the B lymphocyte system of mammals cannot be obtained until the induction site for this line is clearly identified.

Recent evidence indicates that the antibody-forming precursor cells (AFPC) of bone marrow are differentiated to the stage of commitment to antigen. Unanue *et al.* (1971) demonstrated that the bone marrow of unimmunized mice contains cells which bind radiolabeled antigen via immunoglobulin-like cell surface receptors. Moreover, incubation of marrow cells with heavily labeled antigen abolished the capacity of those cells to adaptively transfer humoral response to that particular antigen (Unanue *et al.*, 1971). The demonstration that the precursors of direct and indirect plaque-forming cells can be separated by centrifugation on an albumin gradient constitutes further evidence for commitment of bone marrow AFPC (Miller and Cudkowicz, 1971). Antigen-binding cells bearing membrane-bound immunoglobulins which can now be considered AFPC are found in other lymphoid tissues of unimmunized animals as well (Unanue *et al.*, 1971; Davie and Paul, 1971). These results suggest that there may be no *qualitative* difference in bone marrow AFPC and antigen-binding B lymphocytes in spleen or lymph nodes of unimmunized animals. The synergism observed between bone marrow and thymic or thoracic duct lymphocytes in humoral responses to thymic-dependent antigens, which has led to the concept that the bone marrow is the primary source of AFPC, could be explained by a deficiency of thymic-dependent lymphocytes in this site. In fact, the bone marrow of mice contains relatively few thymic-dependent cells, as defined by the presence of the θ antigen (Raff and Owen, 1971). Further, marrow is a poor source of cells mediating graft *vs.* host reactions (Cantor *et al.*, 1970).

In unimmunized chickens, antigen-binding B lymphocytes are found in peripheral lymphoid tissues. Cells binding the antigen dinitrophenyl guinea pig albumin have been demonstrated in peripheral blood and spleen. The binding is inhibitable by DNP-lysine and by antibodies to chicken immunoglobulin (Davie and Kincade, personal communication). These cells resemble, at least in surface properties, the AFPC of mice. That these cells originate in the bursa of Fabricius has been clearly demonstrated by experiments involving early bursectomy (Kincade *et al.*, 1971; Rabellino and Grey, 1971). We maintain that the same type of experimental data is needed for direct identification of the origin of B lymphocytes in mammals. The presence of AFPC in a particular organ, even if they are the predominant lymphoid cell type, does not constitute evidence for their origin in that site. We conclude that the experimental data in mice provide no positive support for the concept that *differentiation* of uncommitted stem cells to committed precursors of antibody-forming cells occurs in the bone marrow. The fact that the marrow is a repository for both populations is entirely compatible with the GALT theory.

Despite certain critical gaps in the available experimental evidence, we conclude that a large body of circumstantial evidence decidedly favors the concept that lymphoid follicles of GALT are sites in which lymphoid differentiation is induced along plasma cell lines in mammals. At the very least, the GALT hypothesis has focused attention on the paucity of knowledge about lymphoid tissues along the intestines of mammals and has stimulated experimental efforts to correct this deficit. In this regard it has been a useful hypothesis. On the other hand, the most that could have been expected from this hypothesis was that it would help locate the sites in which development along plasma cell lines begins in mammals and, by analogy to the avian bursa of Fabricius, suggest ways of defining their inductive functions. In another review in this volume, we have attempted to point out ways in which study of these induction sites could provide information on the mechanisms responsible for generation of antibody heterogeneity.

REFERENCES

Abdou, N. I., and Richter, M., 1970. Cells involved in the immune response. XVIII. Potential hemolysin-forming cells in the sacculus rotundus of the normal adult rabbit. *J. Immunol.* **104**:1087.

Ackerman, G. A., 1966. The origin of the lymphocytes in the appendix and tonsil iliaca of the embryonic and neonatal rabbit. *Anat. Rec.* **154**:21.

Adler, W. H., Curry, J. H., and Smith, R. T., 1967. Quantitative aspects of early postnatal immunoglobulin polypeptide chain synthesis in the rabbit. In Smith, R. T., Good, R. A., and Miescher, P. A., eds., *Ontogeny of Immunity,* University of Florida Press, Gainesville, p. 165.

Archer, O. K., Sutherland, D. E. R., and Good, R. A., 1963. Appendix of the rabbit: A homologue of the bursa in the chicken? *Nature* **200**:337.

Archer, O. K., Sutherland, D. E. R., and Good, R. A., 1964. The developmental biology of lymphoid tissue in the rabbit: Consideration of the role of thymus and appendix. *Lab. Invest.* **13**:259.

Aspinall, R. L., Meyer, R. K., Graetzer, M. A., and Wolfe, H. R., 1963. Effect of thymectomy and bursectomy on the survival of skin homografts in chickens. *J. Immunol.* **90**:872.

Astaldi, G., Airo, R., Galimberti, A., and Nervi, M. P., (1968). Phytohemagglutinin and human appendiceal lymphocytes. *Lancet* **ii**:172.

Bienenstock, J., and Dolezel, J., 1971. Peyer's patches: Lack of specific antibody-containing cells after oral and parenteral immunization. *J. Immunol.* **106**:938.

Bockman, D. E., and Cooper, M. D., 1971. Fine structural analysis of pinocytosis in lymphoid follicle-associated epithelium in chick bursa and rabbit appendix. *Fed. Proc.* **30**:511, abst.

Brody, T., and Hencin, R., 1969. The immune competence of Peyer's patch cells. *Fed. Proc.* **28**:309, abst.

Cantor, H., Mandel, M. A., and Asofsky, R., 1970. Studies of thoracic duct lymphocytes of mice. II. A quantitative comparison of the capacity of thoracic duct lymphocytes and other lymphoid cells to induce graft *vs.* host reactions. *J. Immunol.* **104**:409.

Chang, T. S., Rheims, M. S., and Winter, A. R., 1957. The significance of the bursa of Fabricius in antibody production in chickens. I. Age of chickens. *Poultry Sci.* **36**:735.

Chapman, H., Johnson, J., and Cooper, M. D. Ontogeny of immunoglobulin-containing cells and gut-associated lymphoid tissue in the pig. Submitted for publication.

Claman, H. N., Chaperon, E. A., and Triplett, R. F., 1966. Thymus-marrow cell combinations—synergism in antibody production. *Proc. Soc. Exptl. Biol. Med.* **122**:1167.

Clawson, C. C., Cooper, M. D., and Good, R. A., 1967. Lymphocyte fine structure in the bursa of Fabricius, the thymus, and the germinal centers. *Lab. Invest.* **16**:407.

Cooper, G. N., and Turner, K., 1967. Immunological responses in rats following antigenic stimulation of Peyer's patches. I. Characteristics of the primary response. *Aust. J. Exptl. Biol. Med. Sci.* 45:363.

Cooper, G. N., and Turner, K., 1969. Development of IgM memory in rats after antigenic stimulation of Peyer's patches. *J. Retic. Soc.* 6:419.

Cooper, M. D., Peterson, R. D. A., and Good, R. A., 1965. Delineation of the thymic and bursal lymphoid systems in the chicken. *Nature* 205:143.

Cooper, M. D., Peterson, R. D. A., South, M. A., and Good, R. A., 1966a. The functions of the thymus system and the bursa system in the chicken. *J. Exptl. Med.* 123:75.

Cooper, M. D., Schwartz, M. M., and Good, R. A., 1966b. Restoration of gamma globulin production in agammaglobulinemic chickens. *Science* 151:471.

Cooper, M. D., Perey, D. Y., McKneally, M. F., Gabrielsen, A. E., Sutherland, D. E. R., and Good, R. A., 1966c. A mammalian equivalent of the avian bursa of Fabricius. *Lancet* I:1388.

Cooper, M. D., Perey, D. Y. E., Gabrielsen, A. E., Dent, P. B., Cain, W. A., and Good, R. A., 1967. Further evidence that Peyer's patch tissues of mammals are similar to the bursa of Fabricius of birds. *Fed. Proc.* 26:752.

Cooper, M. D., Perey, D. Y., Gabrielsen, A. E., Sutherland, D. E. R., McKneally, M. F., and Good, R. A., 1968. Production of an antibody deficiency syndrome in rabbits by neonatal removal of organized intestinal lymphoid tissues. *Internat. Arch. Allergy* 33:65.

Coppola, E. D., DeLuca, F., Kopycinski, C., and Aboul-Enein, A., 1970. Synergistic effect of Peyer's patches and spleen cells on humoral antibody production. *Fed. Proc.* 29:700, abst.

Crabb, E. D., and Kelsall, M. A., 1940. Organization of the mucosa and lymphatic structures in the rabbit appendix. *J. Morphol.* 67:351.

Daguillard, F., and Richter, M., 1970. Cells involved in the immune response. XVI. The response of immune rabbit cells to phytohemagglutinin, antigen, and goat anti-rabbit immunoglobulin antiserum. *J. Exptl. Med.* 131:119.

Davie, J. M., and Paul, W. E., 1971. Antigen binding lymphocyte of non-immune guinea pigs: Specificity and immunoglobulin nature of their receptors. *Fed. Proc.* 30:587.

Davies, A. J. S., 1969. The thymus and the cellular basis of immunity. *Transplant. Rev.* 1:43.

Davies, A. J. S., Leuchars, E., Wallis, V., Marchant, R., and Elliot, E. V., 1967. The failure of thymus-derived cells to produce antibody. *Transplantation* 5:222.

Dent, P. B., and Good, R. A., 1965. Absence of antibody production in the bursa of Fabricius. *Nature* 207:491.

DeSousa, M. A. B., Parrott, D. M. V., and Pantelouris, E. M., 1969. The lymphoid tissues in mice with congenital aplasia of the thymus. *Clin. Exptl. Immunol.* 4:637.

DiGeorge, A. M., 1965. Discussion of paper by M. D. Cooper *et al. J. Pediat.* 67:907.

DiGeorge, A. M., 1968. Congenital absence of the thymus and its immunologic consequences: Concurrence with congenital hypoparathyroidism. In Bergsma, D., and Good, R. A., eds., *Immunologic Deficiency Diseases in Man,* The National Foundation, New York, p. 116.

Evans, E. P., Ogden, D. A., Ford, C. E., and Micklem, H. S., 1967. Repopulation of Peyer's patches in mice. *Nature* 216:36.

Faulk, W. P., McCormick, J. N., Goodman, J. R., Yoffey, J. M., and Fudenberg, H. H., 1970. Peyer's patches: Morphologic studies. *Cell. Immunol.* 1:500.

Friedenstein, A., and Goncharenko, I., 1965. Morphological evidence of immunological relationships in the lymphoid tissue of rabbit appendix. *Nature* 206:1115.

Gilmour, D. G., Theis, G. A., and Thorbecke, G. J., 1970. Transfer of antibody production with cells from bursa of Fabricius. *J. Exptl. Med.* 132:134.

Gitlin, D., 1971. Development and metabolism of the immune globulins. In Kagan, B. M., and Stiehm, E. R., eds., *Immunologic Incompetence,* Year Book Medical Publishers, Inc., Chicago, p. 3.

Glick, G., Chang, T. S., and Jaap, R. G., 1956. The bursa of Fabricius and antibody production. *Poultry Sci.* 35:224.

Good, R. A., and Gabrielsen, A. E., eds., 1964. *The Thymus in Immunobiology,* Hoeber-Harper, New York.

Good, R. A., Cain, W. A., Perey, D. Y., Dent, P. B., Meuwissen, H. J., Rodney, G. E., and Cooper, M. D., 1969. Studies on the nature of germinal centers. In Fiore-Donati, L., and Hanna, M. G., Jr., eds., *Advances in Experimental Medicine and Biology, Vol. 5: Lymphatic Tissue and Germinal Centers in Immune Response,* Plenum Press, New York, p. 33.

Gowans, J. L., and Knight, E. J., 1964. The route of recirculation of lymphocytes in the rat. *Proc. Royal Soc. Lond. B* 159:257.

Hanaoka, M., and Waksman, B. H., 1970. Appendix and γM-antibody formation. II. Distribution of antibody-forming cells after injection of bovine γglobulin in irradiated, appendix-shielded rabbits. *Cell. Immunol.* 1:316.

Hanaoka, M., Konda, S., and Takiguchi, T., 1967. Histological appearance of lymph nodes of rabbits after thymectomy or appendectomy at birth followed by X-irradiation and injection of antigens. *Acta Haematol. Japan* 30:69.

Hanaoka, M., Nomoto, K., and Waksman, B. H., 1970. Appendix and γM-antibody formation. I. Immune response and tolerance to bovine γglobulin in irradiated, appendix-shielded rabbits. *J. Immunol.* 104:616.

Hanaoka, M., Williams, R. M., and Waksman, B. H., 1971. Appendix and γM antibody formation. III. Uptake and distribution of soluble or alum-precipitated bovine γ-globulin injected into the rabbit appendix. *Lab. Invest.* 24:31.

Heim, L. R., McGarry, M. P., and Montgomery, J. R., 1970. Histologic and immunologic capacities of parental spleen, lymph node and Peyer's patch cells in irradiated hybrid mice. *Fed. Proc.* 29:827.

Henry, C., Faulk, W. P., Kuhn, L., Yoffey, J. M., and Fudenberg, H. H., 1970. Peyer's patches: Immunologic studies. *J. Exptl. Med.* 131:1200.

Jacobson, L. O., Robson, M. J., and Marks, E. K., 1950. The effect of X-irradiation on antibody formation. *Proc. Soc. Exptl. Biol. Med.* 75:145.

Jacobson, L. O., Marks, E. K., Simmons, E. L., and Gaston, E. O., 1961. Immune response in irradiated mice with Peyer's patch shielding. *Proc. Soc. Exptl. Biol. Med.* 108:487.

Janković, B. D., and Isvaneski, M., 1963. Experimental allergic encephalomyelitis in thymectomized, bursectomized and normal chickens. *Internat. Arch. Allergy* 23:188.

Janković, B. D., and Mitrović, K., 1967. Antibody-producing cells in the chicken, as observed by fluorescent antibody technique. *Folia Biol.* 13:406.

Kincade, P. W., Lawton, A. R., and Cooper, M. D., 1971. Restriction of surface immunoglobulin determinants to lymphocytes of the plasma cell line. *J. Immunol.* 106:1421.

Konda, S., and Takiguchi, T., 1967. Immune response and changes in gamma globulins in thymectomized and/or appendectomized rabbits. *Acta Haematol. Jap.* 30:85.

Konda, S., and Harris, T. N., 1966. Effect of appendectomy and of thymectomy, with X-irradiation, on the production of antibodies to two protein antigens in young rabbits. *J. Immunol.* 97:805.

Lawton, A. R., Aldrete, J., Mage, R. G., and Cooper, M. D. Manuscript in preparation.

Matsaniotis, N., Apostolopoulou, E., and Vlachos, J., 1966. Thymic alymphocytosis. Report of a case with normal Peyer's patches. *J. Pediat.* 69:576.

Matsumura, T., Noro, Y., Nakomoto, Y., and Miyazaki, F., 1968. Development of the lymphoid cell system in human fetus. XII. Internat. Congr. Pediat., Mexico City, abst.

Meuwissen, H. J., Kaplan, G. T., Perey, D. Y., and Good, R. A., 1969*a*. Role of rabbit gut-associated lymphoid tissue in cell replication. The follicular cortex as primary germinative site. *Proc. Soc. Exptl. Biol. Med.* 130:300.

Meuwissen, H. J., Gatti, M. D., Teraski, P. I., Hong, R., and Good, R. A., 1969b. Treatment of lymphopenic hypogammaglobulinemia and bone marrow aplasia by transplantation of allogeneic marrow. *New Engl. J. Med.* 281:691.

Micklem, H. S., Ford, C. E., Evans, E. P., and Gray, J., 1966. Interrelationships of myeoloid and lymphoid cells: Studies with chromosome-marked cells transfused into lethally irradiated mice. *Proc. Royal Soc. Lond. B* 165:78.

Miller, H. C., and Cudkowicz, G., 1971. Density gradient reparation of marrow cells restricted for antibody class. *Science* 171:913.

Miller, J., 1966. Immunological competence: Alteration by whole body X-irradiation and shielding of selected lymphoid tissues. *Science* 151:1395.

Miller, J. F. A. P., and Mitchell, G. F., 1969. Thymus and antigen-reactive cells. *Transplant. Rev.* 1:3.

Mitchell, G. F., and Miller, J. F. A. P., 1968. Cell to cell interaction in the immune response. II. The source of hemolysin-forming cells in irradiated mice given bone marrow and thymus or thoracic duct lymphocytes. *J. Exptl. Med.* 128:821.

Perey, D. Y. E., and Good, R. A., 1968. Experimental arrest and induction of lymphoid development in intestinal lymphoepithelial tissues of rabbits. *Lab. Invest.* 18:15.

Perey, D. Y. E., Cooper, M. D., and Good, R. A., 1968. Lymphoepithelial tissues of the intestine and differentiation of antibody production. *Science* 161:265.

Perey, D. Y. E., Cooper, M. D., and Good, R. A., 1968. The mammalian homologue of the avian bursa of Fabricius: I. Neonatal extirpation of Peyer's patch-type lymphoepithelial tissues in rabbits: Method and inhibition of development of humoral immunity. *Surgery* 64:614.

Perey, D. Y. E., Frommel, D., Hong, R., and Good, R. A., 1970. The mammalian homologue of the avian bursa of Fabricius. II. Extirpation, lethal X-irradiation and reconstitution in rabbits. Effects on humoral immune responses, immunoglobulins and lymphoid tissues. *Lab. Invest.* 22:212.

Peterson, R. D. A., Cooper, M. D., and Good, R. A., 1965. The pathogenesis of immunologic deficiency diseases. *Am. J. Med.* 38:579.

Pollard, M., and Sharon, N., 1970. Responses of the Peyer's patches in germ-free mice to antigenic stimulation. *Inf. and Immunity* 2:96.

Rabellino, E., and Grey, H. M., 1971. Immunoglobulins on the surface of lymphocytes. III. Bursal origin of surface immunoglobulins on chicken lymphocytes. *J. Immunol.* 106:1418.

Raff, M. C., and Owen, J. J. T., 1971. Thymus-derived lymphocytes: Their distribution and role in the development of peripheral lymphoid tissues of the mouse. *Europ. J. Immunol.* 1:27.

Rubin, E., 1971. The kinetics of cellular proliferation in the bursa of Fabricius. Master's thesis, University of Alabama in Birmingham, manuscript in preparation.

Schultz, R. D., Dunne, H. W., and Heist, C. E., 1970. Ontogeny of the bovine immune response. *Fed. Proc.* 29:699.

Shimizu, Y., and Andrew, W., 1967. Studies on the rabbit appendix. I. Lymphocyte-epithelial relations and the transport of bacteria from lumen to lymphoid nodule. *J. Morphol.* 123:231.

Silverstein, A. M., and Prendergast, R. A., 1971. The maturation of lymphoid tissue structure and function in ontogeny. In Lindahl-Kiessling, K., Alm, G., and Hanna, M. G., Jr., eds., *Advances in Experimental Medicine and Biology, Vol. 12: Morphological and Functional Aspects of Immunity,* Plenum Press, New York-London, p. 37.

Stramignoni, A., and Mollo, F., 1968. Development of the lymphoid tissue in the rabbit's appendix. A light and electron microscopic study. *Acta Anat.* 70:202.

Stramignoni, A., Mollo, F., Rua, S., and Palestro, G., 1969. Development of the lymphoid tissue in the rabbit appendix isolated from the intestinal tract. *J. Pathol.* 99:265.

Stutman, O., and Good, R. A., 1971. Immunocompetence of embryonic hemopoietic cells after traffic to thymus. *Transplant. Proc.* 3:923.

Sussdorf, D. H., 1959. Quantitative changes in the white and red pulp of the spleen during hemolysin formation in X-irradiated and nonirradiated rabbits. *J. Inf. Dis.* 105:238.

Sussdorf, D. H., 1960. Repopulation of the spleen of X-irradiated rabbits by tritium-labeled lymphoid cells of the shielded appendix. *J. Inf. Dis.* 107:108.

Süssdorf, D: H., and Draper, L. R., 1956. The primary hemolysin response in rabbits following shielding from X-rays or X-irradiation of the spleen, appendix, liver or hind legs. *J. Inf. Dis.* 99:129.

Sutherland, D. E. R., Archer, O. K., and Good, R. A., 1964. Role of the appendix in development of immunologic capacity. *Proc. Soc. Exptl. Biol. Med.* 115:673.

Sutherland, D. E. R., McKneally, M. F., Kellum, M. J., and Good, R. A., 1970. A definition of thymic-dependent areas in the peripheral lymphoid tissues of rabbits. *Internat. Arch. Allergy* 38:6.

Thompson, J. H., and Cooper, M. D., 1971. Functional deficiency of autologous implants of the bursa of Fabricius in chickens. *Transplantation* 11:71.

Thorbecke, G. J., 1960. Gamma-globulin formation and antibody production *in vitro*. I. Gamma-globulin formation in tissues from immature and normal adult rabbits. *J. Exptl. Med.* 112:279.

Tyan, M. L., and Herzenberg, L. A., 1968. Studies on the ontogeny of the mouse immune systems: II. Immunoglobulin-producing cells. *J. Immunol.* 101:446.

Unanue, E. R., Grey, H. M., and Cerottini, J. C., 1971. Interaction of lymphocytes and macrophages with radioactive protein antigens. *Fed. Proc.* 30:588.

Warner, N. L., Szenberg, A., and Burnet, F. M., 1962. The immunological role of different lymphoid organs in the chicken. *Aust. J. Exptl. Biol. Med. Sci.* 40:373.

Chapter 4

C3-Receptor Sites on Leukocytes: Possible Role in Opsonization and in the Immune Response

Victor Nussenzweig* and **Carolyn S. Pincus**

Department of Pathology
New York University School of Medicine
New York, New York

INTRODUCTION

In recent years the membrane of lymphocytes has been the subject of intensive study by immunologists, geneticists, and cell biologists. The reasons for this interest are multiple. For example, lymphoid cells can be readily obtained in suspension and in relatively large numbers. They may constitute a model for problems of cellular recognition and differentiation, since they may acquire and lose membrane markers during differentiation (Boyse and Old, 1969; Takahashi *et al.*, 1970; Owen and Raff, 1970), and furthermore, in contact with antigen and other substances, they may be induced to proliferate *in vitro*. For the immunologist, the plasma membrane of lymphocytes is of particular interest because it may contain the specific recognition unit which, after interaction with the antigen, triggers the immunological process (and also the synthesis and/or release of other substances, specific or nonspecific, some of which are mediators of the inflammatory process; Lawrence and Landy, 1969). In addition, the plasma membrane of lymphocytes, as we shall see, bears the markers which allow for their separation into subpopulations which probably have distinct functions in the immune response.

This work was supported by National Institutes of Health Grant AI-08499 and Training Grant AI-00392-02.
* Career Scientist of the Health Research Council of the City of New York, Contract I-558.

RECEPTORS FOR IMMUNOGLOBULIN AND COMPLEMENT
ON MOUSE LEUKOCYTES

A few years ago, Dr. W. Lay and one of us (Nussenzweig *et al.*, 1969; Lay and Nussenzweig, 1968, 1969) started to study the properties of receptors for immunoglobulins (Ig) and complement (C) components on the membrane of leukocytes. The method which we used to detect these receptor sites consisted of allowing close contact between mouse leukocytes obtained from different organs and sheep erythrocytes (E) which had been sensitized with different classes of antibody (A) and complement (C) components. The presence of a specific receptor was ascertained by the formation of clusters or rosettes between the sensitized erythrocytes (EA or EAC) and leukocytes, and these clusters were then counted under the microscope. Some of the results of our experiments are summarized in Table I. Specific receptors for Ig (7S and 19S) and C components (C3, as discussed below) were detected among several types of leukocytes, including lymphocytes. Operationally, these receptors could be readily distinguished from each other. The binding of antigen Ag-19S antibody complexes (Ag-Ab 19S) to macrophages was found to be Ca^{2+}-dependent and could even be reverted when Ca^{2+} was diluted out or chelated with Na_3HEDTA. In contrast, the complement (C3) dependent binding of immune complexes to macrophages, monocytes, and polymorphonuclear (PMN) cells (but not to lymphocytes) was Mg^{2+}-dependent. Also, the receptors for neither Ag-Ab 7S or Ag-Ab 19S were destroyed by trypsin, but treatment with this enzyme appeared to destroy the C3 receptors.

One important point was that serum (or normal 7S Ig) competitively inhibited the binding of Ag-Ab 7S to leukocytes, but did not affect the binding of Ag-Ab-C. This finding supports the idea that C components might play a more important role than 7S antibody in opsonization *in vivo*, since, in most circumstances, this must take place in the presence of "normal" Ig. Also, a large number of C3 sites can be generated on the target cell after a single antigen-antibody site is formed on its surface. We are referring to the known fact that, when antibody binds to a red cell and after it interacts with C1, C4, and C2, the EAC142 complex catalyzes the binding of several hundred C3 molecules to the erythrocyte membrane (Mayer, 1970; Müller-Eberhard, 1968). In this way, the destruction or further handling of a particle or cell which has been recognized as foreign by circulating antibody can be performed by specialized cells which have a receptor for modified C3, such as macrophages, monocytes, PMN cells, and certain lymphocytes (complement-receptor lymphocytes or CRL). This may actually be the reason why the C3 receptor is so widely distributed among leukocytes of all mammalian species tested. In addition, because complement activity is characterized in many of its steps by proteolysis and appearance on the C components of previously unexposed (new) configurations, it generates specific signals of the encounter between antigen and antibody which may subsequently induce leukocyte activity. The native C components present in serum, of course, do not bear these configurations and do not compete for the sites on leukocyte membranes. In other words, from the physiological point of view, a receptor for modified C components appears to be ideally suited for the detection of antigen-antibody interactions, because on the one hand it would never bind antigen or antibody alone, and on the other, through the fixation of C, it would bind the product of the union of most Ag and Ab, independent of their specificities.

DO LYMPHOCYTES SPECIFICALLY RECOGNIZE ANTIGEN-ANTIBODY INTERACTIONS?

In the following section we shall discuss recent evidence showing that bone marrow-derived, thymus-independent (B) lymphocytes may specifically recognize antigen-antibody interactions which have led to complement fixation, since these lymphocytes have a receptor for modified C3 on their membranes. However, this might not be the *only* mechanism through which mixtures of antigen and antibody can induce changes in nonsensitized lymphocytes. In some instances, as we shall point out below, immune complexes appear to stimulate certain lymphocyte functions *in vitro* without a demonstrable participation of C components.

Cytotoxic Function of Lymphocytes

The careful studies of Perlmann and his collaborators (Perlmann and Holm, 1969; Perlmann and Perlmann, 1970) suggest that lymphocytes may recognize IgG either alone or complexed with antigen. They observed that Cr^{51}-labeled chicken erythrocytes were lysed when incubated in culture with purified human peripheral blood lymphocytes, in the presence of heat-inactivated rabbit anti-chicken erythrocyte antiserum. The lysis was optimal with a high ratio of lymphocytes to target cells (20:1), and maximum effects were obtained only after 48 hr of incubation. (This may indicate that under the conditions of the test, the process is not very efficient, or that other factors have to be either synthesized or modified during the incubation period in order to start the reaction.) The possibility that some of the anti-chicken erythrocyte antibody might be cytophilic for lymphocytes appeared unlikely, because purified rabbit IgG inhibited the reaction only when added to the tissue culture medium in very high concentrations, in contrast to what has been observed for antibodies cytophilic for macrophages, monocytes, or PMN.

Also, immunoadherence between antibody-bearing chicken erythrocytes and human lymphocytes was not noticed, and mixed aggregation between lymphocytes and target cells was never a predominant feature in the culture. (This is in agreement with our observations—Lay and Nussenzweig, 1968—that EA cells, prepared with relatively high concentrations of mouse 7S or 19S antisheep red blood cell antibodies, were never found to adhere to mouse lymphocytes.) Participation of complement components in the initial interaction between sensitized chicken erythrocytes and human lymphocytes was not formally ruled out. However, all sera used had been heat-inactivated, and the cytotoxic reaction apparently was not inhibited by rabbit anti-human C3 antiserum. In order to explain his observations, Perlmann suggests that lymphocytes may have a receptor for an immunoglobulin molecule which has suffered a conformational change after contact with antigen. In this respect, it is pertinent to point out that Phillips-Quagliata *et al.* (1971) could not find any such allosteric change in immune complexes which could be recognized by rabbit peritoneal macrophages. In a different system involving the cytotoxic action of immune lymphocytes from sheep on xenogeneic lymphoid target cells, the participation of complement components was strongly suggested by the recent observations of Grant *et al.* (1970). They showed that, under certain conditions, the cytotoxic activity of immune lymphoid cells was increased up to 40 times in the presence of fresh serum, whereas the addition of heat-inactivated serum had no enhancing effect. Moreover, when immune lymphocytes were added at a ratio of 100 or more for each target lymphoma cell, the addition of fresh serum was unnecessary for the cytotoxic reaction, which suggests that lymphoid cells and perhaps some contaminating macrophages (Stecher and Thorbecke, 1967; Rubin *et al.*, 1971) might contain or produce some components of the complement system.

Induction of DNA Synthesis in Normal Lymphocyte Cultures by Antigen–Antibody Complexes

Möller (1969) and Bloch-Shtacher *et al.* (1968) observed that mixtures of antigen and antibodies of various types stimulate nonsensitized lymphocytes to an increased DNA synthesis. The species origin of the antibody did not influence stimulation, but particulate antigens were more efficient than soluble antigens. Maximum stimulation of DNA synthesis occurred rather late, after about 5-6 days of incubation. As Möller (1969) pointed out, although addition of complement to the system did not increase stimulation further, it could not be excluded that certain C components were necessary for the reaction, since they might have been produced by the lymphocytes during the prolonged incubation period. Actually, Bloch-Shtacher *et al.* (1968) noticed an enhancing effect of fresh *vs.* old serum on the rate of DNA synthesis of human lymphocytes in the presence of antigen-antibody complexes.

Antibody-Mediated Immune Suppression of the Immune Response *In Vitro*

The findings of Feldmann and Diener (1970) and Diener and Feldmann (1970) that *in vitro* immune suppression can be mediated by low doses of antigen in the presence of specific antibody may be quite pertinent to this discussion. They showed that an optimal antigen-antibody ratio was required for this "tolerance" induction and that this effect appeared to be central, that is, on the lymphoid cells rather than on the antigen. One interesting point was that an antigen (fragment A of flagellin), which by itself failed to induce tolerance *in vitro*, became effective provided that lymphoid cells were exposed to it for some time in the presence of specific antibody.

In short, at present there seems to be no direct evidence that, in the absence of complement, lymphocytes bind immunoglobulin or antigen-antibody complexes to their membranes. However, it appears certain that lymphocytes, when cultured in the presence of immune complexes, undergo changes which may be secondarily detected as discussed above.

PRESENCE OF A RECEPTOR FOR C3 ON THE MEMBRANE
OF CERTAIN LYMPHOCYTES (CRL)

Most of the work referred to in this section was the result of our collaboration with Drs. Celso Bianco, Peter Dukor, and Aline Eden. The initial observation, referred to previously (see Table I), was that lymphocytes from peripheral lymph nodes, spleen, and thoracic duct of the mouse, but not from its thymus, bound EAC to their membranes, and this of course suggested that they might constitute a separate population of cells. Recent evidence has confirmed this idea and has shown that these lymphocytes (CRL) comprehend most or all B lymphocytes and do not contain or contain very few thymus-derived (T) lymphocytes. The reasons for this statement are as follows: (1) CRL cells are absent from the mouse thymus and present in variable proportion among lymphocytes from different lymphoid organs (Lay and Nussenzweig, 1968; Bianco *et al.*, 1970). Their distribution complements that of θ-bearing cells (T cells) and coincides with that of cells bearing immunoglobulin determinants on their membrane (B cells?) (Bianco *et al.*, 1971). (2) CRL cells localize histologically in the thymus-independent areas of the lymphoid organs (Dukor *et al.*, 1970). (3) An increased proportion of CRL cells are present in lymphoid organs of neonatally thymectomized animals or in lymphoid organs

Table I. Receptors for Immunoglobulins and Complement Factor(s) on Mouse Leukocytes

Receptor for	Cells in which it has been detected	Effect of trypsin treatment of leukocytes	Dependence on divalent cations for binding
7S-immunoglobulin	Peritoneal macrophages, PMN, and blood monocytes	Not affected	Not dependent
19S-immunoglobulin	Peritoneal macrophages	Not affected	Dependent on Ca^{2+}
Complement A	Lymph node and thoracic duct lymphocytes, but not thymus lymphocytes	Destroyed	Not dependent
Complement B	Peritoneal macrophages, PMN, and blood	Destroyed	Dependent on Mg^{2+}

of adult mice which have been thymectomized, X-irradiated, and reconstituted with normal bone marrow. These CRL cells were proven to be of donor origin (Dukor *et al.*, 1971). (4) *In vitro* depletion of CRL cells from a population of lymphoid cells leads to a simultaneous depletion of Ig-bearing cells and enrichment of θ-bearing cells (Bianco *et al.*, 1970; Bianco and Nussenzweig, 1971). (5) *In vitro* depletion of θ-bearing cells from a population of lymphoid cells leads to a relative increase in the proportion of CRL among the remaining cells (Bianco and Nussenzweig, 1971).

For these reasons, we feel that it is warranted to equate the known properties of mouse CRL (Bianco *et al.*, 1970) with the properties of most (or all) B lymphocytes. According to our findings, these mouse B lymphocytes (1) are relatively less dense than T lymphocytes; (2) adhere more readily than T lymphocytes to nylon wool; (3) bear immunoglobulin determinants, but not θ antigen, on their membranes; (4) bear a receptor for a modified C component (C3) on their membranes; and (5) can be either long- or short-lived. To our knowledge this is the first demonstration that B lymphocytes can be long-lived cells. This is of particular interest because B cells also circulate (they are found in the lymph, in the blood, and in the lymphoid organs) and bear immunoglobulin on their membranes. Thus they display properties which are suited for carrying out the functions of antigen-reactive cells and memory cells.

Complement Components Involved in the Interaction Between EAC and CRL

The interaction between EAC and CRL probably involves a split product of C3 which is bound to the erythrocyte membrane, because (Lay and Nussenzweig, 1968; Bianco *et al.*, 1970; Eden *et al.*, 1971); (1) EAC43 but not EAC4 cells (prepared with purified human C components) bind to CRL. (2) EAC cells prepared with complement from C5-deficient mice or C6-deficient rabbits bind as effectively to CRL as EAC prepared with C from normal mice. This observation renders unlikely the participation of the late complement components. (3) Mouse complement, after treatment with cobra venom (which inactivates C3), is ineffective in sensitizing EA for rosette formation with CRL. (4) Rabbit antibodies directed against mouse C3 effectively inhibit and revert the interaction between EAC and CRL. (This finding constituted the basis for the development of a method for the purification of CRL from a mixed population of cells as discussed below.)

The idea that native C3 is not involved, and that a new configuration must be present on C3 for its binding to CRL to occur, is in agreement with the observation that EAC-CRL clusters may be formed in the presence of normal mouse serum which contains a relatively high concentration of native C3. The C3 split product involved is probably C3b. It is known that the EAC42a complex activates C3 and enables it to react with a specific receptor on the red cell membrane. The C3-derived fragments from guinea pig complement have been only incompletely characterized (Mayer *et al.*, 1967). C3 bound to EAC42a is associated with peptidase activity, and it would be of interest to determine its effect on CRL after the interaction occurs.

Nature of the Receptor Site on CRL

Very little is known about the site on the membrane of CRL which binds to modified C3. It may be a protein, since it is destroyed by trypsin treatment (Bianco *et al.*, 1970). Because these C3 receptors may coexist with Ig molecules (Bianco *et al.*, 1970) on the membrane of the same cell, it is possible that the Ig molecules *are* the C3 receptors. This could be conceived in two distinct ways: either the C3 receptor would actually be a cell-bound anti-C3 antibody (immunoconglutinin?), or cell-bound Ig would have the property of interacting with C3b. The first possibility is not very attractive since it would imply that all or most B lymphocytes are synthesizing anti-C3 antibodies. A few arguments can also be raised against the second hypothesis. For instance, as serum Ig does not inhibit the binding of EAC to CRL (in other words, serum Ig apparently does not bind C3b), it would be necessary to postulate a different set of properties for membrane-bound Ig. In addition, we have demonstrated that mouse lymphocytes can be treated *in vitro* with rabbit anti-mouse Ig antibody without affecting their capacity to bind EAC (Bianco and Nussenzweig, 1971). Although none of these arguments is decisive, at present we prefer to consider that C3 receptors and Ig molecules are found at separate locations on CRL membranes.

Specific Isolation of CRL: Properties of the Isolated Population of Cells

The possibility of inhibiting and reverting cluster formation between EAC and CRL by anti-C3 antibodies was the basis for the development of a method to purify CRL from a mixed population of cells (Eden *et al.*, 1971). When clusters of EAC-CRL are treated with papain fragments of rabbit anti-C3 antibodies for approximately 1 hr at 37 C, the erythrocytes come off the surface of the lymphocytes. (Papain fragments of anti-C3 antibody are used in order to avoid agglutination of EAC cells, which have accessible C3 molecules on their surface.) The degree of reversion was shown to be dependent on the concentration of the antibody fragments and on the time (but not temperature) of incubation. For example, 50% reversion was obtained in less than 15 min when the concentration of papain fragments was about 400 μg/ml, but it took 60 min when the concentration of the fragments was 40 μg/ml. Also, the inhibition of rosette formation between EAC and CRL was shown to be dependent on the concentration of EAC. When more C3-sensitized erythrocytes were present, more anti-C3 antibody was needed to achieve a certain degree of inhibition. This is, of course, what would be expected assuming that anti-C3 antibodies and CRL receptor sites compete for the same target, that is, C3 molecules bound to the red cell membrane.

These results imply that the interaction between EAC and CRL is reversible under the conditions tested. However, no spontaneous reversion of EAC-CRL clusters has been observed when these clusters are shaken or incubated for prolonged periods of time at 37°C or 0°C. It is possible that the stability of rosettes in the absence of anti-C3 antibodies is due to the cooperative effect of multiple C3 sites on the erythrocyte binding to multiple receptors on the lymphocyte membrane.

The method for specifically isolating CRL, which was based on these observations, can be summarized as follows: (1) A mixed population of lymphocytes is incubated with EAC to induce the formation of EAC-CRL rosettes. (2) Rosettes are then separated from free erythrocytes and free lymphocytes by the method described by Miller and Phillips (1969), which consists simply of the sedimentation of these particles of different dimensions at 1 g in a bovine serum albumin (BSA) gradient. The velocity of sedimentation was shown by these investigators to be proportional to the radius of the particle. (Thus rosettes, being larger, will sediment faster than free cells.) The actual equipment used for this separation is shown in Fig. 1. It consists of a gradient maker, a peristaltic pump, and a funnel of adequate dimensions. After 2-3 hr of sedimentation of the cells in the funnel, fractions are collected and those containing only or mostly rosettes are pooled. About 20-40% of the rosettes initially present can be recovered with a degree of purity around 95%. (3) The isolated clusters are then treated with anti-C3 antibodies in order to dissociate EAC from CRL. (4) Finally, the erythrocytes are removed by differential flotation in a discontinuous BSA gradient. The supernatant contains purified CRL, and the final recoveries vary from 15 to 30% of the CRL present in the original mixture. Purified preparations of CRL obtained from the mouse spleen were examined for the presence on their membranes of bound immunoglobulins (which are perhaps markers of B cells; Raff et al., 1970; Rabellino et al., 1971a,b) and of the θ antigen (marker of T cells; Reif and Allen, 1964; Raff, 1969, 1970; Schlesinger and Yron, 1970). As expected, 90% or more had membrane-bound Ig and none had θ as could be detected by cytotoxic tests with specific antisera and rabbit complement. This finding, together with previous observations (Reif and Allen, 1964; Raff, 1969, 1970; Schlesinger and Yron, 1970), validates the use of the θ marker for identifying

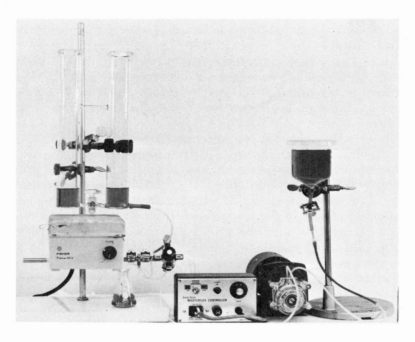

Figure 1. Apparatus used for the purification of CRL. Left: gradient maker. Center: variable-speed peristaltic pump. Right: glass sedimentation funnel. A three-way valve was used to select the fluid to be admitted into the funnel (BSA solution or cell suspension) and at the same time to avoid air bubbles.

thymus-derived lymphocytes. Also, it seems probable that a similar method may be utilized to isolate B cells from other species, in view of our previous observation that lymphocytes from rabbit, guinea pig, and rat also bind EAC and form rosettes (Bianco *et al.*, 1970).

Role of CRL in the Phenomenon of Follicular Localization of Antigen

When antigen is injected into an animal in the presence of small amounts of circulating antibody, it localizes and can be shown to remain for long periods of time in lymphoid organs (Mitchell and Abbot, 1965; Ada *et al.*, 1967; Hanna *et al.*, 1967, 1968; McDevitt *et al.*, 1966; Hanna and Hunter, 1971). This distribution of antigen is far from random and it includes the follicular areas, which contain B lymphocytes (Dukor *et al.*, 1970; Parrott *et al.*, 1966). In view of the prolonged persistence of antigen in these areas and its absence in tolerant animals (McDevitt *et al.*, 1966), it is generally assumed that this phenomenon may be the cellular representation of one of the important events in the immune response, that is, concentration of antigen in a strategic position in lymphoid organs.

For some time, it was thought that the antigen in the follicles was only bound to the membrane of certain reticular cells (present in these areas) whose processes are in intimate contact with the membrane of the neighboring lymphocytes. However, our findings strongly suggest that (1) lymphocytes play a role in this phenomenon and (2) the binding of antigen to the membrane of lymphocytes and dendritic reticular cells is mediated through the C3 receptor. The supporting evidence can be summarized as follows. The follicular localization of antigen is an antibody-mediated phenomenon (Ada *et al.*, 1967; McDevitt *et al.*, 1966; Hanna *et al.*, 1967, 1968; Nossal *et al.*, 1965; Humphrey and Frank, 1967). It is enhanced by passively administered antibody with an intact Fc fragment, but not by F(ab')$_2$ fragments (Ada *et al.*, 1967). As the Fc fragment also mediates C fixation, participation of C components seems possible. Furthermore, aggregated γ-globulin, which effectively binds C, localizes in the follicles (Ada *et al.*, 1964*a,b*). Participation of lymphocytes in the phenomenon is suggested by the observation that the areas in which antigens localize coincide with the areas of distribution of CRL (B) lymphocytes, which of course can bind Ag-Ab-C complexes. Direct binding of antigens to the membranes of lymphocytes and of dendritic reticular cells in the same areas has actually been observed (Dukor *et al.*, 1970). The findings that depletion of lymphocytes by thoracic duct drainage reduces the uptake of antigenic material in those areas and that passive administration of antibody only partially restores localization (Williams, 1966) are in agreement with our hypothesis. Quite relevant also are the recent findings of Brown *et al.* (1970). They incubated mouse lymphocytes with radioactively labeled aggregated human γ-globulin *in vitro* in the presence of serum at 4 C and, after washing the cells, injected them into syngeneic recipients. Immunofluorescence showed that about 40% of these washed cells had the labeled IgG on their surface and that after intravenous injection the labeled antigen could be found in the spleen follicles. Moreover, when these spleens were teased into single cell suspensions and stained for human Ig with specific antisera conjugated with fluorescein, many fluorescent lymphocytes were detected.

Also, Zatz and Lance (1971) recently reported that lymphocytes are "trapped" in the spleen following intravenous and intraperitoneal antigen administration, and in draining lymph nodes following subcutaneous antigen administration or challenge with foreign skin. Such trapping was found in mice undergoing both primary and secondary responses and was antigen dose-dependent. The specificity of this phenomenon was suggested by the fact that lymphocyte trapping can be elicited in presensitized recipients at lower antigen doses than in nonsensitized recipients, and by an accelerated tempo for trapping in secondary allograft responses as compared to primary allograft responses.

Thus, from this evidence it appears possible that immune complexes contribute to the concentration of B lymphocytes in certain areas of the lymphoid organs, where they accumulate around the processes of dendritic reticular cells, thereby forming follicles. As both B lymphocytes and presumably dendritic reticular cells have receptors for modified C3, this complement component may constitute a molecular bridge between these cells. This then could be the explanation at the molecular level of the growth of follicles upon antigenic stimulation. Under these circumstances and because the reaction between the C3 membrane receptor and the immune complexes is reversible, the areas where B lymphocytes accumulate should contain high concentrations of both bound and free antigen. This would of course increase the probability of an encounter between a *specific* antigen-reactive cell present in the follicle and the antigen, particularly during the secondary response or even during a primary response, when natural antibodies are present. This concept is in agreement with the frequent observation that small amounts of antibody can enhance antibody production (Uhr and Möller, 1968).

However, because antibody appears to be also capable of suppressing the immune response to those antigenic determinants which it covers, the net result of antigenic stimulation in the presence of antibody may be the resultant of these opposing effects. When small amounts of antibody are present, the stimulatory effect may predominate and this may be one of the reasons for the vigor of secondary responses. In the next section, we give some recent evidence that the enhancing effect of antibody can be demonstrated at the antigenic determinant level, and moreover that it appears also to be dependent on the Fc fragment of the antibody for full expression.

ENHANCING EFFECT OF ANTIBODY STUDIED AT THE ANTIGENIC DETERMINANT LEVEL

The ability of passively administered antibody specific for one portion of a protein molecule to enhance antibody formation against the determinants of the remaining uncovered region was initially investigated in rabbits immunized with guinea pig γ_2-immunoglobulin and simultaneously receiving passive rabbit anti-guinea pig $F(ab')_2$ antiserum (Pincus and Nussenzweig, 1969). The resulting suppression of the immune response against the $F(ab')_2$ portion of the antigen, detectable early in the immune response, was accompanied at a later time by a significant increase in antibody formation against the adjacent Fc region. When the dose of anti-$F(ab')_2$ antibody administered was varied

(Pincus *et al.*, 1971), it became evident that the enhancement effect was not dependent upon the simultaneous discernible suppression of the response to other determinants on the same molecule (Fig. 2); i.e., whereas suppression of anti-F(ab')$_2$ antibody synthesis was obtained only with large doses of passive antibody (60 mg, 12 mg), enhancement of the anti-Fc response occurred over a wider range of doses (60, 12, 2.4 mg), including that too small to cause suppression of the anti-F(ab')$_2$ response (2.4 mg). In fact, the 2.4 mg dose appeared to augment anti-F(ab')$_2$, as well as anti-Fc, antibody formation, but this increase in anti-F(ab')$_2$ antibody production was not statistically significant at the 5% level ($0.05 < P < 0.10$, at day 35).

Our desire to confirm and extend these findings in an independent yet analogous antigen-antibody system led to the choice as antigen of human secretory immunoglobulin A (IgA), which contains a and L chains like those in serum IgA plus an additional moiety, the weakly immunogenic (Bistani and Tomasi, 1970) secretory component, which is not present in serum IgA

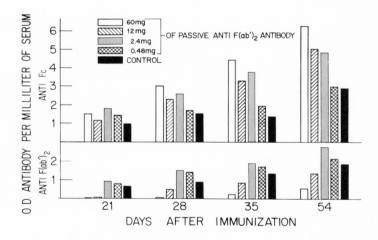

Figure 2. Antibody produced after active immunization with guinea pig γ_2-immunoglobulin by rabbits receiving different amounts of passive anti-F(ab')$_2$ antibody. All rabbits were immunized with 0.5 mg of purified guinea pig γ_2-immunoglobulin incorporated in complete Freund's adjuvant. In addition, they received either rabbit anti-F(ab')$_2$ antibody or normal rabbit serum (controls), administered through several intravenous injectons. At 35 days after immunization, anti-Fc antibody production by groups receiving 60, 12, or 2.4 mg antibody was significantly enhanced in relation to the control group ($P < 0.01, < 0.05, < 0.05$, respectively, Student t-test). Anti-F(ab')$_2$ antibody synthesis at day 35 by groups receiving 60 or 12 mg antibody was significantly suppressed in relation to the control group ($P < 0.001; 0.05 < P < 0.10$, respectively). (Reproduced from Pincus *et al.*, 1971.)

(Tomasi and Bienenstock, 1968). Through the administration of rabbit antibody specific for serum IgA to rabbits immunized with human secretory IgA, the production of antibody specific for the secretory component was significantly enhanced (more than twice as great), while the response to determinants in common with serum IgA was suppressed (Pincus *et al.*, 1971).

What is the molecular basis of this enhancing effect of passive antibody? In view of contradictory reports attributing the phenomenon to only the γM class of antibody (Henry and Jerne, 1968), or to both the γM and γG classes (Perlman, 1967; Pollack *et al.*, 1968), experiments were performed to investigate the ability of the γG fraction of rabbit anti-guinea pig $F(ab')_2$ antiserum to enhance the immune response against the Fc region of guinea pig γ_2-immunoglobulin. Furthermore, since certain other nonspecific properties of immunoglobulins such as cytophilia and complement fixation are mediated through the Fc region of the antibody molecule, we wanted to determine whether the enhancing effect is also Fc-dependent. In the two experiments performed (Pincus *et al.*, 1971), whole antiserum or the γG-immunoglobulin derived from it (containing equal amounts of anti-$F(ab')_2$ antibody) suppressed anti-$F(ab')_2$ antibody synthesis (Fig. 3) and enhanced the anti-Fc re-

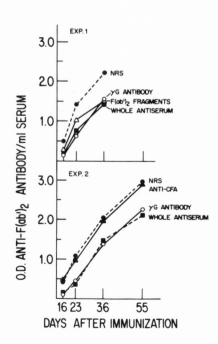

Figure 3. Anti-$F(ab')_2$ antibody produced after active immunization with guinea pig γ_2-immunoglobulin by rabbits receiving passive anti-$F(ab')_2$ antibody in different forms. In both experiments, all rabbits were immunized with 0.5 mg of purified guinea pig γ_2-immunoglobulin incorporated in complete Freund's adjuvant. In addition, in experiment 1 (upper half) two groups of rabbits received a total of 3 mg antibody per animal in either whole anti-$F(ab')_2$ antiserum or purified γG-immunoglobulin, administered through several intravenous injections. The control group received comparable volumes of normal rabbit serum (NRS). Rabbits receiving rabbit $F(ab')_2$ fragments specific for guinea pig $F(ab')_2$ were each injected with a total of 20 mg of antibody fragments. In experiment 2 (lower half) two groups of rabbits received a total of 12 mg antibody per animal in either whole anti-$F(ab')_2$ antiserum or purified γG-immunoglobulin. The rabbits receiving anti-complete Freund's adjuvant (CFA) antiserum or NRS were injected with comparable volumes. (Reproduced from reference Pincus *et al.*, 1971.)

sponse (Fig. 4). Interestingly, the $F(ab')_2$ fragments of the γG antibody also caused suppression of the anti-$F(ab')_2$ response (in accord with the previous findings of Tao and Uhr, 1966; Rowley and Fitch, 1968; Chang *et al.*, 1969; Cerottini *et al.*, 1969), but did not show evidence of having caused enhancement of anti-Fc antibody synthesis at any of the times tested.

These results appear to rule out the possibility of an exclusive role for γM antibody in the enhancement phenomenon (see also Perlman, 1967), although on a molar basis it may prove to be more effective than γG. In addition, from the evidence obtained it appears that the mechanisms for the enhancing and suppressive effects of antibody are unrelated. The timing for achieving maximum suppression or enhancement of antibody formation is not the same (enhancement is only obtained at a later time). Also, enhancement of the response to some determinants may be obtained without discernible suppression of the response to the homologous determinants. Finally, the $F(ab')_2$ fragments of passive antibody can mediate immune suppression but were not observed to enhance the response against the unrelated determinants of the same molecule. It remains to be determined whether the importance of the Fc region for enhancement stems from its role in follicular concentration of antigen, perhaps through complement fixation and subsequent binding of

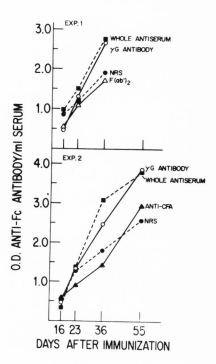

Figure 4. Anti-Fc antibody produced after active immunization with guinea pig γ_2-immunoglobulin by rabbits receiving passive anti-$F(ab')_2$ antibody in different forms. For experimental details, see caption of Fig. 3. (Reproduced from reference Pincus *et al.*, 1971.)

immune complexes to the corresponding complement receptor sites on B lymphocytes and dendritic reticular cells.

CONCLUDING REMARKS

The demonstration of a receptor for modified C3 on the membrane of B lymphocytes evokes some important questions in relation to basic mechanisms in the immune response, because it implies that antigens may enter into contact with lymphoid cells in two distinct ways. First, an antigen may bind to an immunoglobulin receptor or recognition unit on the cell membrane of certain lymphocytes. These cells may proliferate and synthesize antibody which they were precommitted to make. This is, of course, one of the basic postulates of the clonal selection theory, and there is enough experimental evidence to support it. Second, our findings show that complexes of antigen-antibody-complement may adhere to cell membranes through the C3 receptor. In this case the attachment is necessarily nonspecific, and involves *any* B lymphocytes, independently of their precommitment. The consequences of such an encounter are unknown, but from the evidence of Bloch-Shtacher *et al.* (1968), referred to before, it would appear that it may also induce lymphocytes to increase their synthesis of DNA and to divide. If this is confirmed, the question may be raised, for example, whether the frequently observed "nonspecific" increase in immunoglobulin synthesis during an antibody response might not be a consequence of the stimulation of "innocent" bystander B lymphocytes by circulating immune complexes which may be present in the initial stages of the immune response.

ACKNOWLEDGMENTS

We are grateful to Mrs. Gertrude Fastaia for her expert technical assistance.

REFERENCES

Ada, G. L., Nossal, G. J. V., and Pye, J., 1964*a*. *Aust. J. Exptl. Biol. Med. Sci.* **42**:295.
Ada, G. L., Nossal, G. J. V., and Austin, C. M., 1964*b*. *Aust. J. Exptl. Biol. Med. Sci.* **42**:331.
Ada, G. L., Parish, C. R., Nossal, G. J. V., and Abbot, A., 1967. *Cold Spring Harbor Symp. Quant. Biol.* **32**:381.
Bianco, C., and Nussenzweig, V., 1971. *Science* **173**:154.
Bianco, C., Patrick, R., and Nussenzweig, V., 1970. *J. Exptl. Med.* **132**:702.
Bianco, C., Dukor, P., and Nussenzweig, V., 1971. In *Morphological and Functional Aspects of Immunity*, Lindahl-Kiessling *et al.*, eds., Plenum Press, New York, p. 251.

Bistany, T. S., and Tomasi, T. B., Jr., 1970. *Immunochemistry* 7:453.
Bloch-Shtacher, N., Hirschhorn, K., and Uhr, J. W., 1968. *Clin. Exptl. Immunol.* 3:889.
Boyse, E. A., and Old, L. J., 1969. *Ann. Rev. Genet.* 3:269.
Brown, J. C., DeJesus, D. G., and Holborow, E. J., 1970. *Nature* 228:367.
Cerottini, J. C., McConahey, P. J., and Dixon, F. J., 1969. *J. Immunol.* 102:1008.
Chang, H., Schneck, S., Brody, N. I., Deutsch, A., and Siskind, G. W., 1969. *J. Immunol.* 102:37.
Diener, E., and Feldmann, M., 1970. *J. Exptl. Med.* 132:31.
Dukor, P., Bianco, C., and Nussenzweig, V., 1970. *Proc. Natl. Acad. Sci.* 67:991.
Dukor, P., Bianco, C., and Nussenzweig, V., *European J. Immunol.*, in press.
Eden, A., Bianco, C., Nussenzweig, V., *Cell. Immunol.*, in press.
Feldmann, M., and Diener, E., 1970. *J. Exptl. Med.* 131:247.
Grant, C. K., Denham, S., Hall, J. G., and Alexander, P., 1970. *Nature* 227:509.
Hanna, M. G., Jr., and Hunter, R. L., 1971. In Lindahl-Kiessling, K., Alm, G., and Hanna, M. G., Jr., eds., *Morphological and Functional Aspects of Immunity,* Plenum Press, New York, p. 257.
Hanna, M. G., Jr., Makinodan, T., and Fisher, W. D., 1967. In Cottier, H., Odartchenko, N., Schindler, R., and Congdon, C. C., eds., *Germinal Centers in Immune Response,* Springer-Verlag, New York, p. 86.
Hanna, M. G., Jr., Francis, M. W., and Peters, L. C., 1968. *Immunology* 15:75.
Henry, C., and Jerne, N. K., 1968. *J. Exptl. Med.* 128:133.
Humphrey, J. H., and Frank, M. M., 1967. *Immunology* 13:87.
Lawrence, H. S., and Landy, M., eds., 1969. *Mediators of Cellular Immunity,* Academic Press, New York.
Lay, W. H., and Nussenzweig, V., 1968. *J. Exptl. Med.* 128:991.
Lay, W. H., and Nussenzweig, V., 1969. *J. Immunol.* 102:1172.
Mayer, M. M., 1970. *Immunochemistry* 7:485.
Mayer, M. M., Shin, H. S., and Miller, J. A., 1967. *Protides Biol. Fluids* 15:411.
McDevitt, H. O., Askonas, B. A., Humphrey, J. H., Schechter, I., and Sela, M., 1966. *Immunology* 11:337.
Miller, R. G., and Phillips, R. A., 1969. *J. Cell. Physiol.* 73:191.
Mitchell, J., and Abbot, A., 1965. *Nature* 208:500.
Möller, G., 1969. *Clin. Exptl. Immunol.* 4:65.
Müller-Eberhard, H. J., 1968. *Advan. Immunol.* 8:1.
Nossal, G. J. V., Ada, G. L., Austin, C. M., and Pye, J., 1965. *Immunology* 9:349.
Nussenzweig, V., Lay, W. H., and Miescher, P. A., 1969. In Smith, R. T., and Good, R. A., eds., *Cellular Recognition,* Appleton-Century-Crofts, New York, p. 317.
Owen, J. J. T., and Raff, M. C., 1970. *J. Exptl. Med.* 132:1216.
Parrott, D. M. V., deSousa, M. A. B., and East, J., 1966. *J. Immunol.* 123:91.
Pearlman, D. S., 1967. *J. Exptl. Med.* 126:127.
Perlmann, P., and Holm, G., 1969. *Advan. Immunol.* 11:117.
Perlmann, P., and Perlmann, H., 1970. *Cell. Immunol.* 1:300.
Phillips-Quagliata, J. M., Levine, B. B., Quagliata, F., and Uhr, J. W., 1971. *J. Exptl. Med.* 133:589.
Pincus, C., and Nussenzweig, V., 1969. *Nature* 222:594.
Pincus, C., Lamm, M. E., and Nussenzweig, V., 1971. *J. Exptl. Med.* 133:987.
Pollack, W., Gorman, J. G., Hager, H. J., Freda, V. J., and Tripodi, D., 1968. *Transfusion* 8:134.
Rabellino, E., Colon, S., Grey, H. M., and Unanue, E. R., 1971a. *J. Exptl. Med.* 133:156.
Rabellino, E., Grey, H., and Unanue, E., 1971b. *Fed. Proc.* 30:588.
Raff, M. C., 1969. *Nature* 224:378.
Raff, M. C., 1970. *Immunology* 19:637.
Raff, M. C., Sternberg, M., and Taylor, R. B., 1970. *Nature* 225:553.
Reif, A. E., and Allen, J. M. V., 1964. *J. Exptl. Med.* 120:413.

Rowley, D. A., and Fitch, F. W., 1968. In Cinader, B., ed., *Regulation of the Antibody Response,* Charles C Thomas, Publisher, Springfield, Ill., p. 127.

Rubin, D. J., Borsos, T., Rapp, H. J., and Colten, H. R., 1971. *J. Immunol.* 106:295.

Schlesinger, M., and Yron, I., 1970. *J. Immunol.* 104:698.

Stecher, V. J., and Thorbecke, G. J., 1967. *Immunology* 12:475.

Takahashi, T. L., Old, L. J., and Boyse, E. A., 1970. *J. Exptl. Med.* 131:1325.

Tao, T. W., and Uhr, J. W., 1966. *Nature* 212:208.

Tomasi, T. B., Jr., and Bienenstock, J., 1968. *Advan. Immunol.* 9:1.

Uhr, J. W., and Möller, G., 1968. *Advan. Immunol.* 8:81.

Williams, G. M., 1966. *Immunology* 11:475.

Zatz, M. M., and Lance, E. M., 1971. Fed. Proc. 30:409.

Chapter 5

Surface Immunoglobulins on Lymphoid Cells

Noel L. Warner*

Laboratory of Immunogenetics
The Walter and Eliza Hall Institute of Medical Research
Melbourne, Australia

INTRODUCTION

The initiation of an immune response requires the direct interaction of the specific antigen with a lymphocyte. In some immune responses, macrophages play an obligatory role in handling the antigen; in others, this appears not to be necessary (Diener *et al.*, 1970). Selectional theories of immunity (Burnet, 1959) hold that the recognition of antigen is inherent in the responding lymphocyte and that this recognition unit shows the same specificity to antigen as that of the antibody to be produced. The simplest view of this antigen-specific receptor would be that it is in fact the same type of complete antibody molecule as will be eventually secreted by that cell.

Recent studies demonstrating a heterogeneity of lymphocyte types have added further complexities to this problem. This heterogeneity was first strikingly observed in avian studies, in which the bursa-derived population of lymphocytes (B), which are the direct precursors of immunoglobulin-secreting cells, were functionally separated from the thymus-derived population (T) of lymphocytic cells mediating transplantation immunity and delayed hypersensitivity (Warner, 1967; Cooper *et al.*, 1966). This latter population of T lymphocytes functions perfectly well in completely agammaglobulinemic

This is publication number 1543 from the Walter and Eliza Hall Institute. This work was supported by the U.S. Public Health Service Research Grant AM 11234-04, The Australian Research Grants Committee, The Reserve Bank of Australia, and the Chicken Meat Research Council of Australia.
* Senior Research Fellow, N.H.M.R.C. Canberra.

bursaless chickens, which are not capable of synthesizing any detectable complete immunoglobulins even in *in vitro* culture (Warner *et al.*, 1969, 1971). In view of the antigen specificity of T-cell responses, it would again be inferred from selectional theories that the T cell must also have surface antigen-specific receptor inherent to the virgin cell.

Studies in mice have amply confirmed and extended the two-cell lymphocyte classification. Thymus-derived cells were first shown to proliferate specifically in response to antigen without becoming the actual antibody-forming cells (Davies *et al.*, 1967). A collaboration between thymus-derived T cells and bone marrow cells was then shown to lead to antibody production, with the bone marrow providing the precursor of the immunoglobulin (antibody) secreting line (Claman and Chaperon, 1969; Miller and Mitchell, 1969). For the sake of simplicity, the term *B lymphocyte* will be used to cover both bone marrow-derived and bursal-differentiated cells, although formal proof that they are one and the same is still needed.

The phenomenon of carrier specificity of secondary antihapten antibody responses (Ovary and Benacerraf, 1963) has been clearly shown to also involve a cell cooperation between a carrier-specific cell and a hapten-specific cell (Mitchison *et al.*, 1970). The carrier-specific cell was definitively identified to be a T cell (Cheers *et al.*, 1971).

These general considerations on the surface antigen receptor of lymphocytes imply that it is some form of immunoglobulin molecule. The presence of immunoglobulin on the surface of lymphocytes was also strongly implied by a series of studies on the stimulation of blast transformation and DNA synthesis in lymphocyte cultures treated with antiglobulin sera specific for various immunoglobulin class or allotypic antigens (Sell and Asofsky, 1968). These observations have since been basically confirmed in other studies using either cell electrophoresis, immunofluorescence, or autoradiography, and all show the presence of some immunoglobulin on at least some lymphocytes. In this report, a detailed review of all these studies will not be made as it is not intended to be a review. Rather, this report will concentrate on two key questions in this area, and will attempt to discuss our own current approaches to these problems: (1) Is the immunoglobulin detected on the surface of B lymphocytes the actual antigen-binding receptor? (2) Is there immunoglobulin on the surface of T lymphocytes and, if so, of what type, and is it the antigen receptor of these cells? Before considering these two questions in detail, it is essential to stress the recent positive evidence that an antigen-binding receptor is exposed on the surface of both B and T lymphocytes.

EXPRESSION OF *V* GENE IN B LYMPHOCYTES

In the following discussion, it is taken for granted that the ability of an antigen to *specifically* interact with the surface of a lymphoid cell demonstrates the presence of a variable region of at least one immunoglobulin poly-peptide chain, and therefore the expression by that cell of at least one of the immunoglobulin genes coding for a variable region. Whether this is a part or not of a complete immunoglobulin molecule will be discussed later—this section is solely to emphasize that both B and T lymphocytes are expressing, at least, an immunoglobulin variable gene.

The most direct demonstration of antigen-lymphocyte surface interaction is to actually visualize this either by using a very large particulate antigen or by tagging the antigen with an isotope and then visualizing this by autoradiography. The original finding of Naor and Sulitzeanu (1967) was that approximately one out of 1500 mouse spleen lymphocytes would bind ^{125}I-labeled bovine serum albumin. This technique, referred to as detection of antigen-binding cells (ABC), has been extensively studied in four laboratories (Ada et al., 1970; Naor and Sulitzeanu, 1969; Humphrey and Keller, 1970; Dwyer and Mackay, 1971), with basic agreement that this is a technique which is antigen-specific, that it can be blocked by addition of unlabeled specific antigen in excess, that one cell binds only one antigen, and that immune animals show a variable, but often pronounced, increase in numbers of ABC. That at least some of these cells are the precursors of the cells participating in an immune response in vivo to that antigen is indicated by "suicide"-type experiments with very highly radioactive antigens. When spleen cells from unprimed normal mice were incubated in vitro with a very hot flagellin antigen and then washed and transferred to irradiated mice, the ability to respond to a simultaneous injection of that particular antigen was lost, whereas reactivity to a non-cross-reacting flagellin was unaltered (Ada and Byrt, 1969).

Are these ABC of B-lymphocyte or T-lymphocyte type? Several recent lines of evidence strongly indicate that the ABC technique as routinely performed detects primarily, if not exclusively, B cells.

1. Two studies (Naor et al., 1969; Dwyer and Hosking, 1971) of peripheral blood leukocytes from agammaglobulinemic patients showed a marked reduction in numbers of ABC. This is also currently being examined in agammaglobulinemic bursaless chickens, as the human data certainly suggest that these patients lack B cells.

2. Pretreatment of mouse spleen cell suspensions with anti-θ antiserum before application of the labeled antigen showed virtually no difference in numbers of ABC as compared to controls. However, pretreatment with an antiserum specific for B cells reduced the number of ABC by at least 90% (Ada and Raff, unpublished observations). As the θ antigen is a T-cell surface-specific isoantigenic marker (Raff, 1969), these studies strongly infer that T cells are not being detected as ABC.

3. Studies of Basten et al. (1971a) have shown that the B lymphocyte also bears a receptor capable of cytophilically binding immunoglobulins of

several classes through their Fc fragments. Using this property, a method was devised (Basten *et al.*, 1971*b*) for removing B cells from mixed lymphoid populations. Spleen or thoracic duct lymphocytes (TDL) were mixed with a rabbit anti-human γ-globulin (HGG) serum and then passed through a column of beads coated with HGG. In this manner, all cells which had cytophilically bound the antiserum were retained. This included macrophages, granulocytes, and B lymphocytes. When TDL preparations were passed through these columns, the population of lymphocytes that passed directly through was enriched for θ-positive cells and totally lacked B cells, as shown by absence of cytophilic binding of antigen-antibody complexes. When such a population was then examined for direct ABC using ^{125}I fowl γ-globulin (FγG), no ABC were detected (Basten, unpublished observations).

4. Probably the most direct evidence that the ABC technique detects B lymphocytes comes from the study of congenitally athymic mice. This strain carries a recessive autosomal gene nude (*nu nu*) that determines total absence of hair, some defects in salivary glands, and complete and permanent failure of thymic development (Pantelouris, 1968). These mice are completely devoid of θ-positive cells and are incapable of rejecting allogeneic skin grafts and of making antibodies to thymus-dependent antigens such as heterologous erythrocytes (Rygaard, 1969). In recent studies in our laboratory, however, it has been found that these mice are perfectly normal in their ability to make antibodies to *Brucella* antigen, and serum immunoglobulins of IgM and IgG classes are approximately normal in amount. There may be some specific defect in IgA synthesis, and this is presently under investigation. The spleen cells from an 8-week-old *nu nu* mouse were compared with normal CBA spleen cells and with the spleen cells from a 6-week-old CBA neonatally thymectomized mouse for their ability to bind several ^{125}I-labeled antigens in the ABC technique (Dwyer *et al.*, 1971*a*). The results are given in Table I. It is quite apparent that normal numbers of ABC are present in the *nu nu* mouse. This is even more significant than the similar result with the neonatally thymectomized mouse, as such mice are claimed to have some residual θ-positive cells. These results are now being extended to other *nu nu* mice, but with even one example of normal numbers of ABC in a totally T lymphocyte-deficient animal, it is evident that the majority, if not all, of ABC are B lymphocytes.

5. A more indirect piece of evidence has recently been obtained in a study on the nature of the genetic control of the inability of some mouse strains to develop a persisting IgG antibody response to the synthetic antigen TGAL (a copolymer of amino acids Tyr, Glu, Ala, Lys). Whereas C57 mice make a strong antibody response after TGAL immunization in Freund's adjuvant, CBA mice do not (McDevitt and Benacerraf, 1969). Recent studies have shown, however, that when these strains are compared for their ability to

Table I. Antigen-Binding Cells in Athymic Mice[a]

Source of splenic lymphocytes	ABC per 10^4 lymphocytes			
	FLA	HCY	TGAL	DNPBSA
Normal CBA	3.2	11.2	14.5	21.0
Nu nu[b]	3.9	10.2	18.5	16.4
NNTX CBA[c]	3.4	9.4	nt[d]	nt

[a] Antigens used were S. adelaide flagellin (FLA), Hemocyanin (HCY), copolymer Tyr, Glu, Ala, Lys (TGAL), and dinitrophenylated bovine serum albumin (DNPBSA). All mice used were 6-8 weeks of age.

[b] Congenitally athymic nude mice.

[c] Neonatally thymectomized CBA mice.

[d] nt: not tested.

elicit a 4-5 day primary IgM antibody response to TGAL, similar antibody production is found (Warner and Mason, 1971). This early IgM response was also observed in neonatally thymectomized "responder"-strain mice (Grumet et al., personal communication), whereas neither the thymectomized "responder" strain nor the control "nonresponder" strain can persist in the antibody response to reach a strong IgG antibody level. It therefore appears that the early IgM response is thymus-independent and is a result of antigenic stimulation of B cells. The defect in "nonresponders" is therefore a T-cell defect which results in an inability of T cells to collaborate and therefore to promulgate a persisting antibody response. We have accordingly tested mice of several strains for their content of ABC to ^{125}I-TGAL. The results in Table II show that absolutely no difference in ABC numbers is observed in splenic lymphocytes from these strains, which in turn is also consistent with the argument that this technique as presently performed detects only B lymphocytes.

6. In a direct comparison of avian embryonic bursal and thymic cells by the ABC technique (Dwyer and Warner, 1971), only very small numbers were observed in the thymus, whereas large numbers of ABC were found in the bursa, even within only a few days of entry of hematopoietic stem cells into the bursa. This result would apparently imply that the process of differentiation of B lymphocytes from stem cells, which is occurring under the influence of a bursal epithelial factor, involves the activation of both immunoglobulin variable- and constant-region genes (Warner, 1971a; Kincade et al., 1970).

Table II. Antigen-Binding Cells to TGAL in Responder and Nonresponder Mice[a]

Source of splenic lymphocytes	Responder status	ABC per 10^4 lymphocytes
C57Bl	Responder	8.9, 10.7, 16.5
129/J	Responder	13.0
CBA/H	Nonresponder	13.6, 13.6, 16.4
C3H	Nonresponder	12.7
NZC	Nonresponder	8.0

[a] All mice were 6-10 weeks of age. Each value is for an individual spleen cell suspension. Responder status is based on immune response after primary TGAL in Freund's adjuvant and soluble TGAL boosting.

Specific antigen-B cell interaction has also been demonstrated by hapten inhibition, antigen column binding, tolerance, and memory. Thus, Mitchison (1967) showed that the presence of free hapten would inhibit hapten-primed cells (now known to be B cells) from forming antibodies in a cell transfer system. Wigzell and Makela (1970) have shown that specific B lymphocytes are removed on passage through antigen-coated columns without removal of B cells of other specificities. Cell collaboration between B cells and T cells has been shown (Chiller *et al.*, 1970) not to occur if the B cells are derived from tolerant animals. In a test of memory function in B cells (Miller and Sprent, 1971), primed T cells were transferred into irradiated hosts with B cells from either primed or unprimed mice; whereas large numbers of plaque-forming cells resulted in the case of primed B cells, the unprimed B cells were unable to enhance the response of primed T cells even when large numbers of cells were used.

EXPRESSION OF *V* GENE IN T LYMPHOCYTES

As discussed in the previous section, the simplest demonstration of *V*-gene expression (combining site activity) would be the interaction of labeled antigen and cell surfaces. With ^{125}I techniques, this does not appear to readily occur, although with considerably longer exposure times and the use of much higher specific activity antigens this may be possible. The sole exception at present—the presence of significant numbers of ABC in fetal thymus of man and mouse—will be discussed later. Direct interaction of lymphocytes with antigen can also be observed with the rosette technique (Zaalberg, 1964;

Nota *et al.*, 1964) of interaction of lymphocytes and heterologous erythrocytes. While many of the reactive cells in this test are antibody-secreting cells, some appear to be nonsecretors and have only a surface coat of specific antibody. By the use of anti-θ sera, it has been claimed (Greaves and Hogg, 1970) that many of the rosette-forming cells from either normal or immunized mice are θ-positive and are therefore T cells. However, some confusion exists on this point, particularly with the cells of unimmunized mice, as it has also been claimed (Schlesinger, 1970) that these cells are not inhibited by anti-θ pretreatment. Thus, while some doubt must be held regarding the validity of this test as evidence of T-cell interaction with antigen in unprimed populations, most workers in this area agree that a significant proportion of rosette-forming cells from immunized mice are θ-positive.

Specific interaction of antigen with T cells has also been convincingly demonstrated in other systems employing tolerance, memory, or antigen-induced suicide. In similar fashion to the studies with B cells, Chiller *et al.* (1970) induced tolerance to human γ-globulin in mice and showed that thymocytes from these animals would not collaborate with normal bone marrow cells: TDL from mice rendered tolerant to FγG were also not capable of collaborating *in vivo* with B cells in thymectomized irradiated bone marrow-protected recipients, even when coated *in vitro* with FγG by the use of fowl anti-mouse lymphocyte globulin (Miller *et al.*, 1971).

Various studies have demonstrated specific memory in T cells using hapten carrier systems in which it has been shown that the carrier-primed cells are T cells (Mitchison *et al.*, 1970; Cheers *et al.*, 1971). Recent studies (Miller and Sprent, 1971) have also shown that a significant augmentation of the immune response occurs when T cells from primed mice are added to T-depleted TDL and transferred to irradiated recipients. In such a system, although normal T cells can also collaborate, ten times as many cells are required.

Although T cells cannot be readily visualized at present with ^{125}I-labeled antigens, if the specific activity of the iodinated antigen is very high, radiation-induced inactivation of T cells will occur. Thus, when thymus lymphocytes were incubated with high specific activity FγG, then mixed with B cells and transferred to irradiated recipients, inactivation of the immune response to FγG occurred, but not to other antigens such as horse red blood cells (Basten *et al.*, 1971c).

These studies and many others not cited all confirm that B and T cells both have exposed antigen-binding sites on their surfaces which are presumed, at the moment, to represent immunoglobulin *V*-gene expression. That immunoglobulins are also present on the surface of B lymphocytes has been documented in several studies (Sell *et al.*, 1970; Raff, 1970; Rabellino *et al.*, 1970; Pernis *et al.*, 1970), although no clear evidence of the presence of immunoglobulin on the surface of unprimed T cells has appeared. The following sections will examine data from our laboratory relevant to this question and to whether the interaction of antigen with antigen receptor sites on T or B lymphocytes can be interfered with by antiglobulin sera.

BLOCKING OF ABC BY ANTI-IMMUNOGLOBULIN SERA

ABC techniques have demonstrated the presence of antigen combining sites on the surface of B lymphocytes, and immunofluorescent and autoradiographic techniques with antiglobulin sera have shown the presence of both immunoglobulin L and H chains. The essential question is whether these two observations in fact concern one and the same immunoglobulin molecule, i.e., a complete molecule with a variable region, and L and H constant regions. As an approach to this problem, we have attempted to interfere with antigen-lymphocyte interaction by pretreating the lymphocyte with antiglobulin sera and then introducing the labeled antigen. The basic assumption in this approach is that when inhibition of antigen binding occurs, it indicates that the receptor site is in immediate proximity to the immunoglobulin chain recognized by the antiserum and is in fact on that immunoglobulin molecule. The alternative possibility is that the antigen recognition site is separate from, but near to, surface-bound immunoglobulin and that the binding of the anti-immunoglobulin onto the latter causes steric hindrance to antigen attachment. While this cannot be rigorously eliminated, it is most unlikely, because in those situations where it has been examined the same type of immunoglobulin receptor has been found by blocking and synthesis studies.

Specific antisera were raised in rabbits against isolated mouse and human myeloma proteins of all L- and H-chain types and were rendered specific by appropriate immunoabsorption. These were then used at varying concentrations (usually 1:5) to react with lymphoid cell suspensions prior to the addition of labeled antigen. Some of the results from previous studies (Dwyer and Mackay, 1971; Warner *et al.*, 1970) are summarized in Table III. Polyvalent anti-Ig almost completely blocks antigen binding to adult mouse spleen and human peripheral blood lymphocytes. This result would strongly indicate that antigen uptake by these tissues is mediated by a surface immunoglobulin. When monospecific antisera were used, only anti-light chain (κ in mouse, and pooled κ and λ in man) and anti-μ heavy chain would significantly block binding. The mean values given are around 10-30% of control, but in some individual experiments the value was as low as 5% of control, i.e., at least 95% inhibition of antigen binding. These results clearly imply that IgM forms the predominant if not the only surface immunoglobulin receptor on unprimed B lymphocytes. No consistent blocking was observed with other anti-H chain reagents, a range of 0-25% inhibition being observed. As this level of blocking

Table III. Inhibition of Antigen-Binding Cells by Anti-Immunoglobulin Sera

Source of cell suspension	Percent of ABC relative to control (no serum)			
	Polyvalent anti-Ig	Anti-light[a] chain	Anti-μ chain	Other anti-heavy chain
Adult mouse spleen	5	29 (135)[b]	30	89, 107
Adult human peripheral blood	15	3	11	86
Mouse peritoneal exudate	23	nt[c]	nt	nt
Mouse neonatal spleen	29	nt	nt	nt
Human fetal bone marrow	100	nt	nt	nt

[a]Anti-κ for mouse, mixed anti-κ and anti-λ for human.

[b]Anti-κ blocked with κ light chain.

[c]nt: not tested.

is rather marginal, and was not even consistently observed, it is doubtful whether these other classes are really represented on unprimed resting B lymphocytes. As the data are very similar for both man and mouse, using entirely separate sets of reagents, we feel that this strongly reinforces the argument that the majority of unprimed B cells have surface IgM as antigen receptor.

It has also been consistently observed that antigen binding can occur in some cell populations without being mediated by surface immunoglobulin. In mouse peritoneal exudate and neonatal spleen cell suspensions, approximately 20-30% of cells appear to bind antigen without involving an immunoglobulin receptor. In fetal mouse liver and fetal human bone marrow, this in fact accounts for all of the antigen-binding cells. Whether these cells are really lymphocytes is debatable. These cell suspensions all contain many hematopoietic cells which may have other types of receptors for antigens. Alternatively, if they belong to the macrophage or granulocyte precursor series, they may have cytophilically bound a small amount of natural antibody, in which case blocking by antiglobulins would be expected. Perhaps the configurational position of cytophilically bound antibody is rather different than that actually synthesized by the cell and held in the membrane, and is not readily accessible to blocking. This is not a very satisfactory explanation, and further studies on these apparently non-Ig mediated ABC are needed.

As previously reported (Dwyer and Warner, 1971), the ABC in the avian bursa of Fabricius can be considerably inhibited by anti-Ig sera. Although we have not yet performed immunoglobulin class analysis of this blocking, it is most likely that it is due to IgM, as the embryonic bursa (days 14-17) appears only to contain (Kincade *et al.*, 1970) and synthesize (Thorbecke *et al.*, 1968) IgM globulin. Again some ABC were found in this location which could not be blocked by anti-Ig pretreatment, but these only occurred in the lightly labeled category (2790 ABC per 10^6 cells in control, 1350 per 10^6 after anti-Ig) in comparison to virtually complete blocking in the heavily labeled cells (5200 per 10^6 in control, 70 per 10^6 after anti-Ig).

Of considerable interest has been the problem of ABC in the fetal and young adult thymus. Are these really antigen-binding T lymphocytes? Is the mammalian thymus also a bursal equivalent? Are the ABC a small population of infiltrating B lymphocytes? Or are they nonspecific ABC of the type found in fetal liver and bone marrow? Complete resolution of this problem can only be made when double markers for T surface isoantigens and immunoglobulins are concurrently or sequentially applied to the same cells. At present, however, it is clear that the last possibility at least has been excluded, as the ABC in thymus can be completely inhibited by anti-Ig sera pretreatment (Dwyer *et al.*, 1971*b*). The results are summarized in Table IV, and it is notable that similar results were again obtained for man and mouse, as both show blocking with anti-light and anti-μ sera, but not with other anti-heavy chain sera. In man, neither anti-κ nor anti-λ completely blocks, and the sum of the two suggests that both κ IgM and λ IgM cells are present, in approximately the

Table IV. Inhibition of ABC in Fetal and Neonatal Thymus by Antiglobulin Sera

Antiserum pretreatment	Percent inhibition of ABC formation[a]			
	Mouse		Human	
Anti-κ	73, 100, 100	(91)	41, 46, 53, 61, 66	(53)
Anti-λ	nt[b]		40	(40)
Anti-μ	86, 89, 100	(92)	80, 88, 88, 99, 100	(91)
Anti-α	0, 0, 0	(0)	0, 11	(5)
Anti-γ_1[c]	0	(0)	0, 0, 0, 0, 8, 10	(3)
Anti-γ_2	0, 0, 0	(0)		

[a]Percent inhibition relative to control cell with no antiserum pretreatment. Each value is for an individual thymus cell suspension with the mean values given in brackets.

[b]nt: not tested.

[c]For human, anti-γ reacting with all γ classes.

same proportions as in serum immunoglobulins. In mouse, the anti-κ serum gives virtually complete blocking, which is in accord with the observation that approximately 95% of mouse immunoglobulin is κ in type. These results therefore show that ABC in either fetal or young adult thymus have the same IgM receptor as peripheralized B lymphocytes. Whether these indeed represent immigrant peripheral-derived cells, or true T cells, will have to be further resolved. A careful study of peripheralized T cells, such as column-purified TDL and educated T cells should be made.

The implication that T cells may have IgM surface receptors has also been made by Greaves and Hogg (1970) using the rosette-forming cell technique (RFC). In similar fashion to the blocking of ABC by cell pretreatment with anti-Ig sera, RFC formation can be completely inhibited by pretreatment with either anti-light chain or anti-Fab sera. The results with anti-heavy chain sera pretreatment are somewhat more complex, as they are dependent on whether the cells are from immune or normal animals. It was found (Greaves and Hogg, 1970) that only 15% of RFC from unprimed animals could be blocked by anti-μ, whereas up to 76% of RFC from 5 days after immunization could be so blocked. As this latter group contained many θ-positive cells (up to 40%), it was implied that some of these may also have been μ-positive. On passage through cotton filtration, an RFC population which was 85% θ-positive was obtained. This was also 85% inhibitable by some anti-μ sera, by anti-light chain sera, but not by other anti-heavy chain sera. It was therefore suggested that the T cell in the normal unimmunized mouse had a buried μ chain which became exposed on antigenic activation of the cell. The results with other anti-heavy chain sera on the entire RFC population suggested that many of the non-θ-positive RFC (B cells?) had multiple heavy chains on their surface, as the value of percent of rosettes blocked by individual anti-heavy chain sera added up to well over 100%.

There are, however, several confusing aspects about this general approach. Firstly, the identification of T-positive cells in these splenic populations relies solely on the anti-θ serum which is not made between coisogenic mice and accordingly may have some other activities which are not truly T-specific. Furthermore, some of these observations have not been completely confirmed in our laboratory. Two main points emerge from recent studies of Wilson et al. (1971): (1) In unprimed mice, there were few θ-positive RFC, which is in agreement with the data of Schlesinger (1970). Furthermore, 71% of these RFC could be inhibited by anti-μ chain serum, in contrast to the figure of 15% of Greaves and Hogg (1970). As the inhibition by anti-κ is 90%, this would suggest that the large majority of the unprimed RFC are B lymphocytes with IgM receptors. This is also in agreement with a study of Bankhurst and Wilson (1971) which shows that 70% of RFC are also ABC, when the two techniques are simultaneously combined using ^{125}I-labeled FγG and FγG-coated sheep erythrocytes. As this figure is identical to the value for anti-μ inhibitable RFC, and as virtually all ABC are μ-positive, it is very suggestive that the unprimed population of RFC is made up of 70% B cells which are all IgM positive and about 20% θ-positive T cells which are positive only for L chain. (2) Whereas the percent of θ-positive RFC decreased over the 0-9 day postimmunization period in Greaves' study (from 41 to 48% positive at 0 time to 24% at 6 days), Wilson observed a rise from 18% at day 0 to 53% on day 9. At this latter point, the percent of RFC inhibitable by anti-μ remained unchanged at around 70%. However, the values for anti-γ and anti-a have risen, and although the summation of anti-heavy chain values are not nearly as high as those of Greaves and Hogg (1970), they are over 100%. This would apparently again imply pluripotentiality in the heavy-chain expression of single cells. Two alternative explanations could be proposed: (a) that with the production of antibody, cytophilic immunoglobulin has bound to the B cell (Basten et al., 1971a), thus increasing the number of immunoglobulin classes on the cell surface; (b) that if the θ-positive RFC in the immunized animal are always μ-positive (which for our 9-day value must be the case for at least half of the θ-positive cells), then this value of 53% (θ-positive) must be subtracted from the value of 78% (μ-positive) to give the true value of μ-positive B cells. Thus, at this time point (9 days), there are about 25% μ-positive B cells, some of which may be solely μ but others may be multi-heavy chain type. Clearly, various assortments of these data could be made, depending on the proportion of T cells that were to be μ-positive, and, further, more precise data are required.

Thus, although there are some rather marked differences in our RFC data and those of other studies, it is rather inescapable that at least some of the θ-positive RFC from immunized animals have surface IgM receptors and that some of the B cells may have several heavy-chain surface receptors. An interpretation of these data will be given in the concluding section.

BLOCKING OF FUNCTIONAL ACTIVITIES OF T LYMPHOCYTES

In our initial approach to the problem of blocking of functional activities of T lymphocytes (Mason and Warner, 1970), the graft vs. host reaction in mice was used as a model of T-cell "killer" activity. Spleen cell suspensions were incubated in the cold with anti-Ig antisera for 3 hr prior to injection into F1 hybrid mice. With three different antisera, virtually total blocking of the graft vs. host reaction was observed. In one instance where tested, the serum from the rabbit before immunization did not inhibit, and in another case the antiserum did not inhibit when it had been preabsorbed with free light chains.

These sera all had anti-light chain activity, which in one case was the only anti-Ig activity present. On the other hand, it must be pointed out that this inhibition could not be obtained with four other anti-Ig sera, all containing some anti-light chain activity. In preliminary tests, we have also observed inhibition of wasting disease with some sera containing anti-light chain activity, but not with others. As the preimmunization serum of one of the inhibitory antisera did not inhibit the reaction, it must be concluded that immunization of the rabbit with a light-chain preparation produced an antibody which reacts with both light chains and the receptor site of the T cell. If this is indeed a light-chain receptor, why do not all anti-light chain sera inhibit?

Answers to this question are clearly only speculative at this stage, and further investigations are proceeding. It is possible that the inhibitory antisera contain an antibody against a critical region of the light chain which is not in all anti-light chain sera. As blocking of an antigen-specific receptor is involved, a minimal requirement is that the receptor contain a product of a variable-region immunoglobulin gene. In studies with anti-human Bence Jones sera, we have found that by appropriate absorption, some antisera will discriminate between κ light chains of different subgroups as determined by amino acid sequence analysis. This therefore raises the possibility that it is only an anti-variable region antibody that can effectively recognize the T-cell antigen receptor site, and that the noninhibitory anti-light chain antisera only contain anti-light constant region activity. This possibility is clearly open to experimental testing.

If reproducible anti-Ig blocking of T-cell activity is possible, then this opens up a further approach to the problem of eradication of secondary disease in bone marrow transplantation. The goal of this procedure is to effectively implant hematopioetic stem cells without transferring immunocompetent cells which can mount a graft vs. host reaction. In testing our various anti-Ig antisera for nonspecific cytotoxic activity, we used (Warner, 1971b) the hematopoietic stem cell colony-forming assay (Till and McCulloch, 1961) on the same spleen cell suspension that was used for graft vs. host reactions. In all cases, spleen colony counts ranged between 50 and 100% of the control values. A similar observation has also been reported by Tyan (1971). This strongly suggests that anti-Ig sera will not have deleterious effects on stem cell activity, and pretreatment of bone marrow cells with an appropriate anti-light chain serum might therefore offer a rapid and simple approach to elimination of immunocompetent activity.

The cellular transfer of delayed hypersensitivity also offers a stage in which activated T cells are held in vitro and are therefore amenable to pretreatment with anti-Ig sera prior to transfer. Although we have obtained (Mason and Warner, 1970) some inhibition in this test with anti-light chain serum pretreatment, it is not a particularly convenient test, as the transfer reaction in mice is quite weak, and in further studies we have not been able to obtain any clearer results with this system. The main problem is that large numbers of cells must be transferred, and the reaction must be scored histologically for lymphocytic infiltration.

Inhibition of *in vitro* mixed lymphocyte reactions has also been achieved with anti-human light chain globulin (Greaves, 1970). As the anti-Ig is itself stimulatory to lymphocytes, this was performed with the Fab fragment of the antibody. Marked inhibition was observed, and the inhibitory activity could be removed by preabsorption of the antibody fragment with light chains. This again confirms the presence of light chain in the T-cell receptor.

In an attempt to work with purified T-cell suspensions, we have recently investigated (Basten *et al.*, 1971c) the radioactive antigen "suicide" killing of virgin T cells from mouse thymus. The biological test used was to transfer the thymocytes to lethally irradiated mice together with a normal B-cell suspension and antigen. After 15 days, antibody-forming cells were assayed by a plaque technique. As the experimental design required that the T and B cells be allowed to interact, it was important to ensure that opsonization and clearance of the injected cells into the liver did not occur. Accordingly, pepsin-digested $F(ab')_2$ fragments of the antibody globulin were prepared. Normal thymocytes were then pretreated with either the pepsin fragment of normal rabbit IgG or of the IgG of anti-mouse light chain antibody. After incubation and washing, the cells were incubated with a high specific activity preparation of ^{125}I-labeled FγG, or with cold ^{127}I-FγG. After further incubation and washing, the cells were mixed with normal B cells and transferred to irradiated mice given FγG. The specific experimental details are given elsewhere (Basten *et al.*, 1971c). The results (Table V) show that pretreatment with ^{125}I-FγG reduced plaque formation to 3.5% of the control value. The effect was specific, as shown by a normal response to an unrelated antigen. Pretreatment of the T cells with the anti-light chain fragment abolished the suicide effect (88% of control). This clearly indicates that the receptor for the labeled FγG contains a light chain. Further studies are in progress with pepsin fragments of anti-heavy chain antibodies.

Blocking of T-cell activity in primary antibody production *in vitro* has also been demonstrated (Lesley and Dutton, 1970) to occur with anti-κ light chain antibody, which provides further evidence that both collaboration assays and "killer"-cell assays of T-cell function demonstrate κ light chain presence in the antigen receptor site.

The hormonally bursectomized chicken provides a convenient experimental model of an animal which is completely lacking in B cells, as shown by its inability to synthesize IgM or IgG immunoglobulin (Warner *et al.*, 1969). As a prelude to further studies with this animal, we have recently

Table V. Inhibition of ^{125}I FγG-Induced T-Cell Suicide
by Anti-κ Pretreatment[a]

Immunoglobulin pretreatment	Antigen pretreatment	Percent peak 7s PFC/spleen	
		FγG plaques	Horse RBC plaques
Normal rabbit IgG F(ab')$_2$	^{125}I FγG	3.5	122
Anti-κ IgG F(ab')$_2$	^{127}I FγG	102.0	202
Anti-κ IgG F(ab')$_2$	^{125}I FγG	88.0	210

[a] The experimental design involves pretreatment of T cells (thymocytes) with F(ab')$_2$ fragments of IgG followed by incubation with hot or cold iodinated FγG. Washed cells are then transferred into irradiated recipients together with FγG and horse RBC antigenic stimulation. The values give the percent of spleen antibody plaque formation relative to the control normal rabbit IgG F(ab')$_2$ and cold ^{127}I FγG pretreatment.

investigated the graft *vs.* host reaction that is induced on the chorioallantoic membrane (CAM) of chicken embryos by allogeneic adult peripheral leukocytes from normal birds (Rouse and Warner, 1971). Local lesions are produced on the membrane as a result of stimulation of donor cells by host histocompatibility antigens (Boyer, 1960). Specific anti-light chain and anti-heavy chain antisera were prepared in rabbits against chicken immunoglobulins and were used to pretreat normal leukocytes prior to their inoculation onto the CAM. Controls involved pretreatment with either normal rabbit sera, no sera, or the anti-light chain sera preabsorbed with immunoabsorbent bound IgG or light chain. The results from this series are summarized in Table VI. Of several antisera used, including three different anti-light chain sera, only one serum reproducibly inhibited focus formation. This was an antiserum prepared against isolated light chains of normal chicken IgG. Although complete suppression was only occasionally observed, some degree of inhibition was always obtained with this serum. The important control is the demonstration that this inhibitory activity was removed by absorption with purified chicken IgG or light chains.

Although further studies are still proceeding along this line, it is already clear that these results with avian systems, and a new set of anti-immunoglobulin antisera, conform to the previous findings with mouse models, name-

Table VI. Effect of Anti-Light Chain Pretreatment of Adult Fowl Leukocytes
on CAM Focus Formation[a]

Serum pretreatment	Percent of control median focal count	Mean (%)
Rabbit anti-chicken light chain	0, 7, 23, 25, 37, 45, 50, 60, 80	36
Rabbit anti-chicken light chain preabsorbed with chicken IgG	43, 75, 86, 95, 112	82

[a] The individual values show the percent of the median focal count for each experiment (6-10 CAM per group) relative to control balanced salt solution or normal rabbit serum pretreatment.

ly, that although many anti-Ig sera cannot inhibit T-cell activity, when a serum is found to do so, its activity is related to its anti-light chain antibody.

BLOCKING OF FUNCTIONAL ACTIVITIES OF B LYMPHOCYTES

As a measure of functional activity of B lymphocytes, we have studied the ability of normal spleen cell suspensions to transfer antibody production to lethally irradiated syngeneic mice simultaneously injected with antigen. Several antigens have been used, including *Brucella abortus* vaccine (BR), *Salmonella* flagellin polymer (POL), and sheep erythrocytes (SRBC). As antibody production to the first two antigens is completely normal in adult thymectomized lethally irradiated bone marrow-protected mice, and in congenitally athymic nude mice, it can be concluded that the transfer of immune responsiveness to at least these two antigens is solely by virtue of B-cell activity. In the case of SRBC, both T and B activity is required. Attempts to interfere with this transfer of immunity by pretreatment of spleen cells with anti-immunoglobulins have been made in three different ways (Herrod and Warner, 1971): (1) by pretreatment with anti-Ig sera in the presence of complement at 37 C, (2) by pretreatment with high specific activity ^{125}I-labeled purified anti-Ig antibodies, and (3) by pretreatment with anti-Ig sera in the cold for 2 hr followed by immediate injection into recipients.

Numerous attempts have been made with each of these approaches, and at present they might be summarized by saying that significant inhibition has been observed with anti-μ chain sera, but it has never been a complete abolition of the immune response, and it has not always been observed in each experiment. The results are summarized in Table VII, and the following points might be made in relation to the three methods used: (1) No inhibition was observed when the cells were held at 37°C with anti-μ serum and complement prior to transfusion into irradiated recipients. This might possibly indicate that the receptor is constantly being turned over at a rapid rate at 37°C, and accordingly the "blocking" antibody and receptor are coming off the cell without permitting complement fixation to occur. (2) Purified anti-immunoglobulin antibodies were prepared by absorbtion of anti-human IgM sera to bromacetylcellulose-conjugated human IgM. The antibodies were then eluted at low pH and were iodinated to high specific activity with ^{125}I. These

Table VII. Inhibition of Cellular Transfer of Antibody Formation with Anti-μ Treated Unprimed Spleen Cells

Spleen cell pretreatment	Experiment no.	Percent control value[a]			
		CFU	DPFC	EPFC	BR
Anti-μ 37°C and complement	1		115		
	2		110		
Mean			112		
^{125}I IgG of anti-μ	3		24	105	
	4	63	32	79	
	5		17	74	
	6	77	18	33	107
	7	68	49	79	31
	8	70	50	88	54
Mean		69	32	77	64
Anti-μ 2 hr 0°C	9		29	70	8
	10		22	82	16
	11	100	39	110	6
Mean		100	30	87	10

[a] All values are expressed as percent of the control (Eisen's balanced salt solution treatment) for each assay system. Each value represents the percent of control, using mean values for groups of four to eight mice. The assays were performed 5-8 days after the pretreated cells were transferred into lethally irradiated recipients given antigen. The assays performed were the spleen colony assay for hematopoietic stem cells (CFU) (Till and McCulloch, 1961); antibody plaque-forming cells to sheep erythrocytes, with both direct plaques (DPFC) and antiglobulin-enhanced plaques (EPFC); serum agglutinins to *Brucella abortus* (BR).

antibodies show cross-reaction to mouse IgM globulins. Normal spleen cells were treated *in vitro* with these preparations, then washed and injected into irradiated recipients. This experiment is analogous to ^{125}I antigen-induced suicide, but in this case we cannot control for nonspecific radiation damage by the use of another antigen, so instead we have examined for radiation-induced impairment of hematopoietic stem cell activity in the same spleen cell suspension by the colony-forming assay. Although a minor fall in spleen colony count was sometimes observed, it was not as marked as the fall in antibody plaque number. The results with this approach, however, have not been very reproducible or satisfactory, and further studies are proceeding. (3) The clearest demonstration of inhibition of B-cell function by pretreatment with anti-μ chain sera has come from the simple incubation of unprimed spleen cells with antiserum in ice for 3 hr prior to transfusion. The results show a marked fall in both anti-BR response and plaque formation to SRBC, thus confirming the *in vitro* blocking of ABC, which also implies that IgM forms the predominant surface antigen receptor on unprimed B lymphocytes.

This approach of inhibition of the transfer of immune responsiveness by anti-μ chain pretreatment is very relevant to the question of sequential synthesis of IgM and IgG. Using the open carboxymethylcellulose hemolytic plaque technique, it was recently demonstrated (Nossal *et al.*, 1971) that individual cells releasing both IgM- and IgG-specific antibody do exist in the immune population. Using a micromanipulation transfer technique with monolayers containing different anti-immunoglobulin reagents, it was possible to discriminate between direct lytic IgG producers, "breakthrough" IgM producers (non-inhibitable by anti-μ), non-complement fixing IgM, regular IgM producers, regular enhanced IgG producers, and double IgM-IgG producers. Of 900 selected antibody-forming cells examined in either primary or secondary responses, 14 (1.5%) were double producers. This study firmly establishes that specific antibodies of two different heavy-chain types can be released from one cell. However, this still does not prove that these cells are actually in the state of transition from IgM production to IgG production. They may represent a small proportion that are fixed in the double-producing state or represent a small proportion of pluripotential cells that are able to further differentiate into either IgM, or IgA, or IgG producers. If all subsequent IgG producers obligatorily arose from IgM-producing precursors, then it would be expected that pretreatment of the unprimed B population with anti-μ antisera would not only inhibit the subsequent IgM production but also the IgG production. Two experimental approaches to this problem are currently under investigation. In the experiments with anti-μ blocking described in Table VII, we have also examined for the effect on enhanced (IgG) plaque production. The results are rather preliminary, as it has proven to be difficult to obtain good IgG production in the transfer system when using unprimed B cells as donors. Although a better IgG production would result if primed spleen donors were used, this would defeat the purpose of the study, as we must start with anti-μ treatment of the *resting* B cell. At least it can be said, that no clear evidence of IgG suppression has been obtained in experiments where suppression of IgM production was found. A second approach has been the transfer of anti-μ treated normal spleen cells from one strain of mouse to a coisogenic partner strain differing in immunoglobulin allotype. Quantitation of donor-type IgG_2 is made with serum samples taken at various times after transfer, and a significant reduction in donor IgG_2 production has been found. The values of donor IgG_2 in the anti-μ treated group are lower than controls, and further studies are proceeding on this approach.

DIRECT BINDING OF ANTI-IMMUNOGLOBULINS TO B LYMPHOCYTES

The studies of Sell and Asofsky (1968) and Sell *et al.* (1970) and the phenomenon of antiallotype suppression of immunoglobulin synthesis *in vivo* (Herzenberg, 1970; Dray, 1962) both strongly imply that B lymphocytes have surface immunoglobulins. This has also been found by Raff (1970) and Rabellino *et al.* (1970) using fluorescein-conjugated antimouse immunoglobulins, by Pernis *et al.* (1970) with rabbit lymphoid cells, and by Coombs *et al.* (1970) using the mixed antiglobulin reaction. In all cases, these authors were unable to find any labeling of thymus cell suspensions.

Using ^{125}I-labeled IgG fractions of highly specific rabbit anti-mouse light chain and heavy chain antisera, we have examined (Bankhurst and Warner, 1971) various mouse lymphoid cell suspensions by autoradiography, after incubation with the antiglobulins. When lymphoid cell suspensions were incubated with about 4 μg of labeled globulin and the autoradiographs were exposed for 3-7 days, heavily labeled cells were observed in both spleen and TDL suspensions with all antisera used, but only small numbers (maximum 6.3%) were observed in thymus, and only with anti-κ immunoglobulin (Table VIII). In view of this much lower value for thymus than for TDL, and since the TDL value rose to 65% with TDL from neonatally thymectomized mice (known to contain predominantly B cells), it is clear that these conditions almost exclusively label surface immunoglobulins on B lymphocytes. In all cases the binding is specific, and can be inhibited completely either by blocking of the antiglobulin with its specific antigen bound to an immunoabsorbent or by pretreatment of the spleen cells with homologous unlabeled anti-immunoglobulin. The values for κ-positive, γ-positive, and a-positive cells in both spleen and TDL were identical, and respectively averaged 32, 20, and 20%. The values for μ-positive cells were higher for spleen (36%) than for TDL (24%). In the case of TDL, the summation of the individual anti-heavy

Table VIII. Labeling of Mouse Lymphoid Cells with ^{125}I Antiglobulins[a]

^{125}I IgG antiglobulin (3-8 μg)	Percent of labeled cells (3-8 day exposure)			
	Spleen	TDL	Thymus	
Anti-κ	33.0	31.3	3.7	(6.3)[b]
Anti-μ	36.3	23.9	0.3	
Anti-γ$_2$	20.8	20.1	1.0	
Anti-α	22.7	20.6	1.5	
Normal rabbit IgG	0.3	0	0	

[a] Each value is the mean of several experiments with amounts of labeled antiglobulin and exposure times between the above limits.

[b] In one individual experiment, the value of 6.3 was found.

chain values is approximately 64%, which is double the κ value. Since normal TDL cells are approximately 20% θ-negative and approximately 20% B cells, as shown by cytophilic IgG-receptor studies (Basten *et al.*, 1971*a*), the B population in TDL would appear to be virtually all pluripotential for heavy-chain type. Again the possibility that this result is due to *in vivo* bound cytophilic immunoglobulin cannot be entirely dismissed, although these cells have been first washed under conditions which should remove B-cell cytophilic immunoglobulin prior to application of the ^{125}I-labeled reagent. Further studies on this aspect are in progress, using both thymectomized mice and allophenic mice, in an attempt to formally eliminate the cytophilic theory and to confirm whether or not the B cell is pluripotential for different heavy chains and also whether or not it shows allelic exclusion (Sell *et al.*, 1970), which is a definite property of the more mature plasma cell (Warner *et al.*, 1966).

DIRECT BINDING OF ANTI-IMMUNOGLOBULINS TO T LYMPHOCYTES

As mentioned in the preceding section, when anti-immunoglobulins were applied to thymus cell suspensions, no significant labeling was found. However, in our (Bankhurst and Warner, 1971) studies with ^{125}I-labeled reagents, the value for thymus (6%), albeit low, was still appreciably above zero. This suggested the possibility that the actual surface concentration of immunoglobulins on the T cell may be much lower than that on the B cell, and accordingly this lower amount might be more demonstrable either by increasing the specific activity of the ^{125}I-label reagent or by exposing the autoradiographs for considerably longer periods. As the first approach was found not to be practical (due to loss of antibody combining activity), we have studied (Bankhurst *et al.*, 1971*a*) various T-cell suspensions which were treated with the same ^{125}I-labeled antiglobulins, but the autoradiographs have been exposed for 50-60 days. These studies have now provided direct visualization of immunoglobulin on the surface of a large majority of T lymphocytes. The results from several experiments are summarized in Table IX, and show that at least 17% of thymocytes and at least 50% of peripheralized T cells have surface κ light chain. No evidence of surface heavy chain of any type, including μ, was found. That the labeling is due to anti-chain activity is shown by the complete absence of binding with specifically absorbed antiglobulin. This increased value for thymocytes over that given in Table VIII is roughly in proportion to that expected on the ratio of increase in exposure time. This therefore implies that perhaps all T lymphocytes in thymus have surface κ chain, but in a variable concentration, and we are now just beginning to get within the range of detectability. The higher value of 50% was obtained with a population of TDL derived from heavily irradiated F1 hybrid mice given parental thymocytes. This population is known to be entirely of T-lymphocyte type and contains activated T cells against the other parental histocompatibility antigen in the host (Sprent and Miller, 1971). This population has

Table IX. Labeling of Mouse T Cells with ^{125}I Antiglobulins and Long-Term Exposures[a]

^{125}I antiglobulin IgG (6-8 μg)	Percent of labeled cells (54-60 day exposure)			
	Thymus		T.TDL	
Anti-κ	13.7	17.0	19.0	49.0
Anti-κ blocked with κ	nt[b]	0	0	0
Pooled anti-heavy chain	nt	1.3	0.3	1.3
Anti-μ	0.3	nt	0	nt
Anti-γ_2	0	nt	nt	nt
Anti-a	0	nt	nt	nt
Normal rabbit IgG	1.0	nt	nt	nt

[a]Each value is for an individual experiment. The thymus cells were from the thymuses of normal 6-week-old mice, and the T.TDL were TDL derived from (CBA × C57)F$_1$ mice previously injected with CBA thymocytes.

[b]nt: not tested.

been termed T.TDL (Sprent and Miller, 1971). Although accurate grain count data are not yet available on the thymus T $vs.$ the T.TDL population, the percentage of κ-positive cells strongly suggests that antigenic activation of the resting T cell has resulted in an increased density of κ chains on the surface of the T.TDL. It is most notable that in this situation activation has not resulted in IgM-positive T cells, in contrast to the data on RFC (Greaves and Hogg, 1970).

Studies with agammaglobulinemic bursaless chickens (Warner $et\ al.,$ 1969) have shown that many of these birds cannot synthesize complete IgM or IgG globulins, and this would suggest that they have no B cells. Using the same techniques with anti-chicken immunoglobulin reagents labeled with ^{125}I, we have now confirmed (Bankhurst $et\ al.,$ 1971b) that no labeled cells are present in these birds with either anti-κ, anti-μ, or anti-γ reagents, when experiments are carried out under the conditions known to detect only B cells in mice. Prolonged exposures are now being performed on this series in order to determine whether immunoglobulin is also present on the avian T-cell surface. These birds could provide a most suitable model to study effects of antigen priming, etc., on receptor density on T cells.

As all these studies with T cells have indicated an extremely low surface receptor density, a more sensitive approach to this problem has been attempted with an immunoglobulin "sandwich" type of assay system (Nossal $et\ al.,$ unpublished observations). The basic experimental design is to incubate well-washed lymphoid cell suspensions (2×10^6 spleen cells or 5×10^6 thymus cells) in a volume of 0.2 ml with a suitable concentration of whole monospecific rabbit anti-mouse immunoglobulin serum, and after further thorough washing of the cells to add high specific activity ^{125}I-labeled IgG of a sheep anti-rabbit immunoglobulin. After further incubation and washing, a sample of the cells is prepared for autoradiography and another sample for direct counting of radioactivity. A sample of these results are given in Table X. Several points can be made about this approach: (1) Normal rabbit serum in place of the rabbit anti-immunoglobulin sera always gives some positive binding, indicating that a certain level of nonspecific binding is occurring. (2) On spleen, all anti-heavy chain sera give quite marked binding, even at very high dilution of the antiglobulin sera (1:10,000), and this binding is almost totally reduced by specific blocking of the antiglobulin serum. (3) With thymus, however, although binding has been consistently obtained with several different anti-light chain sera, and with one preparation of anti-IgM sera, specific blocking of these sera has considerably reduced but not totally eliminated binding.

The positive statement that can be made at present about thymus in this test is that some antiglobulin sera do bind to thymus and that much of this binding can be eliminated by absorption of the sera with myeloma-bound

Table X. Binding of Antiglobulins to Mouse Thymus Cell Suspensions[a]

Serum	Rabbit anti-mouse immunoglobulin	^{125}I sheep anti-rabbit IgG	Binding of ^{125}I (c.p.s.)	
R14	Anti-κ	+	562	
R14	Anti-κ abs. κ	+	181	(68%)
R19	Anti-κ, μ, γ, a	+	1011	
R19	Anti-μ	+	429	(58%)
R18	Anti-κ, a	+	255	
R18	Anti-a	+	65	(75%)
R16	Anti-κ, γ_2	+	415	
R16	Anti-γ_2	+	126	(70%)

[a] In each experiment, 5×10^6 thymocytes were treated with 1 μl of antiserum in a volume of 200 μl. After incubation and washing, the cells were reacted with an ^{125}I-labeled IgG of sheep anti-rabbit immunoglobulin. After further incubation and washing, the cells were counted. The results are given as counts per second (c.p.s.) for a constant aliquot of cells. The value in brackets represents the percent inhibition of binding in the absorbed vs. unabsorbed serum. All absorptions were made with myeloma-bound polyaminopolystyrene.

immunoabsorbents. Thus, this test also confirms the presence of some type of immunoglobulin on the surface of T lymphocytes. Its exact characterization by this test is not fully clear; as with the use of myeloma proteins, there is the possibility that absorbed sera may still have some type of V_H recognition. Further analysis of this is in progress, and certainly some type of light-chain component is present. Again we have observed in this test system that many anti-Ig sera do not appear to bind and that for a given rabbit anti-immunoglobulin serum that does bind, sequential serum samples from the rabbit taken during a prolonged immunization regime behave somewhat differently. Although anti-light chain precipitating activity increases, binding ability to T cells decreases, perhaps because of a decline in proportion of anti-V_L to anti-C_L activity.

SYNTHESIS OF IMMUNOGLOBULINS BY B AND T CELLS

A basic theoretical problem in this work is that surface immunoglobulin can be derived by either passive absorption from outside of the cell or be actually made by the cell on which it is found. This is not a trivial point, as, for example, some immunoglobulin has been shown (Frommel et al., 1967) to be present on the surface of normal mature erythrocytes, which are certainly not synthesizing immunoglobulin. Therefore, the only ultimate answer to the problem of immunoglobulin gene expression in B and T cells must come from synthesis studies, which actually demonstrate immunoglobulin polypeptide chain synthesis by such markers as incorporation of radioactive amino acids into the surface receptor molecule.

Single-cell studies with normal mouse plasma cells (Marchalonis *et al.*, 1968) have shown that these cells contain and release a homogeneous immunoglobulin. This is also readily demonstrable in malignant forms of this cell series, i.e., plasmacytomas. Although the ideal goal would be to study possible immunoglobulin synthesis in completely purified normal B- and T-cell suspensions, it is reasonable to apply the plasmacytoma parallel to lymphocytes and to study thymomas and lymphomas for immunoglobulin synthesis.

A series of radiation-induced thymomas, spontaneous lymphomas, and oil-induced lymphomas are now being screened for possible immunoglobulin synthesis by the technique of Hochwald *et al.* (1961), using tissue fragments in an 18-24 hr roller tube culture with ^{14}C-amino acids. Some of the results at hand are given in Table XI.

Ten transplanted lines of radiation-induced thymomas have been examined. In six cases, no immunoglobulin synthesis has been detected, and these lines are being further studied with larger amounts of tissue samples.

Table XI. Immunoglobulin Synthesis by Murine Lymphoid Tumors

Tumor line	Origin	Short-term *in vitro* immunoglobulin synthesis
WEHI-2	Spontaneous (NZB × BALB/c)F_1 lymphoma	L chain[a]
WEHI-5	Mineral-oil (NZB × BALB/c)F_1 lymphoma	L chain ? IgM
WEHI-6	Spontaneous (NZB × C57BL)F_1 lymphoma	IgM
WEHI-37	Spontaneous (NZB × C57BL)F_1 lymphoma	L chain[a]
WEHI-7	Radiation-induced BALB/c thymoma	Not detected
WEHI-14	Radiation-induced BALB/c thymoma	Not detected
WEHI-16	Radiation-induced BALB/c thymoma	Not detected
WEHI-20	Radiation-induced BALB/c thymoma	Not detected
WEHI-22	Radiation-induced BALB/c thymoma	IgM
WEHI-26	Radiation-induced BALB/c thymoma	? trace L chain
WEHI-27	Radiation-induced BALB/c thymoma	Not detected
WEHI-31	Radiation-induced BALB/c thymoma	? trace L chain
WEHI-105	Radiation-induced BALB/c thymoma	L chain ?
WEHI-106	Radiation-induced BALB/c thymoma	Not detected

[a] Also confirmed by sucrose gradient centrifugation.

One line, WEHI-22, has been established in permanent culture and has been confirmed to be θ-positive. In short-term culture, IgM synthesis has been shown with this line, although the relative amount of immunoglobulin synthesized is extremely small as compared to plasmacytoma lines. A faint but definite IgM line was observed in 6-week exposed plates of the disrupted cultured cells, but not of the concentrated culture fluid. This would perhaps indicate that the tumor line is synthesizing small amounts of IgM which are not being actively secreted from the cell. In three other lines, faint labeling in the anodal end of the IgG line was observed. From previous observations with this technique, this would indicate free light-chain synthesis. Further studies are now in progress with these lines, using permanent tissue culture lines with tritiated amino acid incorporation and immunoprecipitation techniques.

Four other lymphoma lines which arose as primary tumors in peripheral sites rather than in the thymus have also been investigated. Two are synthesizing and secreting free light chains without any demonstrable heavy-chain synthesis. Sucrose density gradient ultracentrifugation of the supernatant of the culture fluid shows banding of synthesized immunoglobulin in the light-chain region. The other two lines both show IgM synthesis of a more pronounced amount than that observed with WEHI-22 (thymoma), with one of them also showing free light-chain synthesis. Unfortunately, we do not have data on the θ status of these lines, and whether these are malignant B or T cells is unknown. Free light-chain synthesis and secretion are often observed in variant lines of plasma cell tumors which have been in passage for some time. This has been particularly frequent in plasmacytoma lines from NZB or NZB F_1 hybrid mice and includes many lines which for several generations synthesized both light and heavy chains and secreted intact Ig molecules, and then produced a variant line which continued to synthesize and secrete only light chain. Such an event might also occur in lymphoma lines, leading to the type of results observed for WEHI-2 and WEHI-37.

Further studies with this approach are required and must involve isoantigenic markers for B and T cells and preferably use recently produced tumor lines.

IMMUNOGLOBULIN GENE EXPRESSION IN LYMPHOID CELL DIFFERENTIATION

The presence of immunoglobulin and of antigen receptor sites on both T and B cells is now quite firmly established, and in most instances they are also quite clearly one and the same molecule. The major unresolved questions concern the actual nature and number of immunoglobulin classes that are expressed by the cell, when they are expressed in the differentiation of the uncommitted immunocompetent cell, and what effect antigen stimulation of the uncommitted cell has on the type and amount of immunoglobulin synthesized.

An attempt to incorporate most of the available data into a working hypothesis is presented in Fig. 1. The essential points of this diagram and their experimental bases are as follows:

1. The uncommitted B cell arises by differentiation from the hematopoietic stem cell under the inducing influence of the avian bursa of Fabricius and its mammalian equivalent (Warner, 1971*a*). In the process of this differentiation, both immunoglobulin light-chain and μ heavy-chain genes are expressed (including variable-region genes) and a complete IgM molecule is assembled and is secreted at a relatively slow rate. This accounts for much of "natural antibody," and the slow rate of synthesis and secretion allows for a persistent surface-bound IgM which acts as antigen receptor. The strongest evidence relevant to this aspect is the demonstration of synthesis (Thorbecke *et al.*, 1968) and surface presence (Kincade *et al.*, 1970) of *only* IgM in the

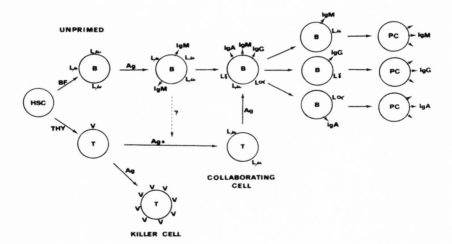

Figure 1. Immunoglobulin expression in lymphoid cell differentiation. It is proposed that a hematopoietic stem cell (HSC) differentiates to a B lymphocyte (B) having IgM receptors (light-chain L and heavy-chain μ) under the influence of the bursa of Fabricius or its equivalent (BF), or to a T lymphocyte (T) under thymic induction (THY). This latter cell expresses only variable-region gene(s) (V). Antigenic (Ag) stimulation of the B cells leads to some IgM antibody release and to activation of other heavy-chain genes (γ, a). Antigenic stimulation of the T cell produces killer cells with increased V-gene activity, or, under the additional influence of activated B cells, to collaborating T cells having IgM surface receptors. These cells collaborate with the pluripotential activated B cells and induce further differentiation to either IgM-, IgA-, or IgG-secreting plasma cells (PC).

embryonic bursa. That this is associated with the emergence of antigen recognition is shown by ABC studies of the bursa (Dwyer and Warner, 1971). The data from the ABC technique in mice, when used under conditions which primarily, if not exclusively, detect B cells, also show only IgM surface receptors. Similar studies with the RFC method on unimmunized spleens have also shown only IgM (Wilson, 1971) for about 70% of the RFC, with the remainder possibly being T cells with only light chains.

2. In similar fashion, the hematopoietic stem cell can also differentiate into a T cell, provided it comes under thymic induction. In this differentiation pathway no constant-region heavy-chain gene is expressed. The exact nature of the immunoglobulin is still uncertain. Our results (Bankhurst *et al.*, 1971a) with direct antiglobulin binding to normal thymocytes have so far indicated only the presence of light chain. However, both in tests with the use of unlabeled antiglobulins followed by iodinated sheep antirabbit globulin (Nossal *et al.*, unpublished observations) and in the blocking of functional activities of T cells, the T-cell binding or inhibitory activity of the antisera has not always exactly followed its immunochemical behavior in liquid precipitation tests. Whether this indicates that only the variable-region gene is expressed, rather than a complete light chain, is still under investigation. In fact, to account for the marked specificity of T-cell combining sites, it may be that both the variable genes for light and heavy chains are expressed, without either of the corresponding constant-region genes.

3. The next stage in differentiation is antigen-induced. In the case of the B cell, it is proposed that direct stimulation of the B cell (with or without macrophage mediation) will result in an increased rate of synthesis of IgM, which therefore leads to the detectable release of some IgM antibody. Probably the clearest evidence relevant to this point is the studies with TGAL. As a second consequence of antigen stimulation, derepression of other constant-region genes occurs, with the result that B cells with multiple heavy-chain types appear in the population. These are detectable by either antiglobulin stimulation (Sell *et al.*, 1970), RFC inhibition (Greaves and Hogg, 1970), or direct antiglobulin binding (Bankhurst and Warner, 1971). The rate of synthesis in all these B cells is still quite low, and further events will now be dependent upon a second factor. This can apparently occur in several ways, because for some antigens it is in the form of a collaborating activated T cell, but for other antigens this is not necessary, and presumably there is something about the form or properties of these antigens that mimics the role of the collaborating T cell. It is therefore proposed that in the presence of excess antigen the now pluripotential B cell is stimulated (via collaborating T cell or some other pathway) to further differentiation toward the end-product goal, namely, a cell whose prime function is to produce a specific protein. These final stages, which involve several more divisions, lead to expression of only

one heavy-chain gene in the end-product cell. Anti-μ blocking of IgG synthesis should therefore only be possible at the unprimed B-cell level (Kincade et al., 1970), and the recent data (Wang et al., 1970) on human myeloma proteins of both IgM and IgG classes present in one individual with identical variable-region genes, but made in different cells, are compatible with this view. The prediction would be that the oncogenic process in this type of patient happened to strike at a differentiating B cell which was somewhere in the pluripotential to next division stage.

4. In the course of this differentiation process from unprimed B cell to mature plasma cell, several other surface markers of B cells change, and accordingly should be further investigated, as they may provide suitable markers for determining the exact stage in differentiation of a particular B cell. These include the loss of the B-cell surface antigenic marker (Raff et al., 1971) the loss of the cytophilic receptor for Fc of immunoglobulins (Basten et al., 1971a), and the acquisition of the PC-1 isoantigenic system (Takahashi et al., 1970).

5. To return to T-cell differentiation, it is envisaged that two alternative pathways exist. The basic proposal is that there are two different types of T cells, and there is indeed in vivo experimental evidence supporting this (Cantor and Asofsky, 1970). Both pathways commence with the unprimed T cell, having perhaps only V-gene expression. Along one path, perhaps induced by free antigenic stimulation, T-cell proliferation occurs, with an increased rate of synthesis, perhaps reflected as increased receptor density of the same variable-region genes but still without any constant-region heavy-chain gene expression. This cell is the "killer cell," mediating transplantation immunity, and may well be the type examined by antiglobulin reagents in the study of Bankhurst et al. (1971), which concerned T.TDL educated in a graft vs. host situation.

6. The alternative pathway is perhaps induced by antigen presented to T cells, not free, but in the form of soluble complexes with IgM or as complexes on B cells (Basten et al., 1971a). This pathway would therefore only occur in situations where the B-cell differentiation pathway had progressed to the stage of liberation of a small amount of antibody. As there is no firm evidence at present on whether or not B cells are needed to permit education of T cells to collaborating cells, this possibility must be considered. It is therefore envisaged that this direction of differentiation results in the T cell expressing both variable-region genes and μ heavy-chain gene. The evidence available at present for this consists solely of the existence of θ-positive RFC in immunized animals and perhaps the θ-positive WEHI-22 thymoma line which syntheses IgM. The problem of ABC in fetal and young adult thymus that can be blocked by anti-μ sera may be relevant to this question, but in the absence of strict confirmation that they are T cells, this cannot be considered as formal evidence. This activated IgM T cell is able to induce further differentiation of the B-cell line, as considered above.

7. The only virtue of attempting to propose all-embracing hypotheses is to predict useful experiments which will confirm, refute, or modify the hypotheses. Probably the main points needing further experimentation are the following: (a) Is the presence of B cells necessary for antigen induction of T cells into "collaborating" cells? (b) Are "killer" cells as defined by suitable assays also "collaborating" cells, and *vice versa*? (c) Will T.TDL educated to a protein antigen such as FγG have both κ and μ surface immunoglobulin, in distinction to graft *vs.* host educated T.TDL cells, which have only κ present? (d) Does the pluripotential B cell really exist, in the sense that it represents intracellular synthesis of several heavy-chain constant regions, each bound to the same specificity variable region? (e) How do some antigens replace the collaborating T cell? (f) Do unprimed T cells synthesize only variable regions, and, if so, are they of light- and/or heavy-chain type?

With the available markers of differentiation of T and B cells and the present wealth of techniques in this field, it is probable that many of these questions will be answered in the relatively near future.

ACKNOWLEDGMENTS

In compiling this analysis of the surface immunoglobulin work, I am most grateful to various colleagues at the Institute, with whom many of these experiments were performed, for their permission to use previously unpublished data. I would like to thank Prof. G. Ada, Drs. A. Bankhurst and A. Basten, Mrs. P. Byrt, Miss P. Crewther, Drs. J. Dwyer and A. Harris, Mr. H. Herrod, Misses H. Lewis and S. Mason, Dr. J. F. A. P. Miller, Prof. G. J. V. Nossal, and Drs. B. Rouse, J. Sprent, and D. Wilson.

REFERENCES

Ada, G. L., and Byrt, P., 1969. *Nature* 222:1291.
Ada, G. L., Byrt, P., Mandel, T., and Warner, N. L., 1970. In Sterzl, J., and Riha, H., eds., *Developmental Aspects of Antibody Formation and Structure,* Academic Press, New York, p. 503.
Bankhurst, A. D., and Warner, N. L., 1971. *J. Immunol.,* in press.
Bankhurst, A. D., Warner, N. L., and Sprent, J., 1971a. *J. Exptl. Med.,* in press.
Bankhurst, A. D., Rouse, B. T., and Warner, N. L. 1971b. *Int. Arch. Allergy,* in press.
Bankhurst, A. D., and Wilson, J., 1971. *Nature,* in press.
Basten, A., Warner, N. L., and Mandel, T., 1971a, manuscript in preparation.
Basten, A. Miller, J. F. A. P., and Sprent, J., 1971b. *Nature,* in press.
Basten, A., Miller, J. F. A. P., Warner, N. L., and Pye, J., 1971c. *Nature,* 231:104.
Boyer, G. S., 1960. *Nature* 185:327.
Burnet, F. M., 1959. *The Clonal Selection Theory of Acquired Immunity,* Cambridge University Press, Cambridge.
Cantor, H., and Asofsky, R., 1970. *J. Exptl. Med.* 131:235.
Cheers, C., Breitner, J., Little, M., and Miller, J. F. A. P., 1971. *Nature,* in press.
Chiller, J. H., Habicht, G. S., and Weigle, W. O., 1970. *Proc. Natl. Acad. Sci.* 65:551.
Claman, H. N., and Chaperon, E. A., 1969. *Transplant. Rev.* 1:92.

Coombs, R., Gurner, B., McConnell, I., and Munro, A., 1970. *Internat. Arch. Allergy* 39:280.
Cooper, M. D., Peterson, R. D. A., South, M. A., and Good, R. A., 1966. *J. Exptl. Med.* 123:75.
Davies, A. J. S., Leuchars, E., Wallis, V., Marchant, R., and Elliot, E. V., 1967. *Transplantation* 5:222.
Diener, E., Shortman, K., and Russel, P., 1970. *Nature* 225:731.
Dray, S., 1962. *Nature* 195:181.
Dwyer, J. M., and Hosking, C. S., 1971. Manuscript in preparation.
Dwyer, J. M., and Mackay, I. R., 1971. *Clin. Exptl. Immunol.,* in press.
Dwyer, J. M., and Warner, N. L., 1971. *Nature, New Biol.* 229:210.
Dwyer, J., Mason, S., Warner, N. L., and Mackay, I. R., 1971a. *Nature,* in press.
Dwyer, J., Warner, N. L., and Mackay, I. R., 1971b. Manuscript in preparation.
Frommel, D., Grob, P. J., Masouredis, S. P., and Isliker, H. C., 1967. *Immunology* 13:501.
Greaves, M. F., 1970. *Transplant. Rev.* 5:45.
Greaves, M. F., and Hogg, N. M., 1971. In Cross, A., Kosunen, T., and Makela, O., eds., *Proceedings of the Third Sigrid Julius Symposium on Cell Cooperation in the Immune Response,* Academic Press, New York, p. 145.
Herrod, H., and Warner, N. L., 1971. *J. Immunol.,* in press.
Herzenberg, L. A., 1970. *J. Cell. Physiol.* 76:303.
Hochwald, G. M., Thorbecke, G. J., and Asofsky, R., 1961. *J. Exptl. Med.* 114:459.
Humphrey, J. H., and Keller, H. U., 1970. In Sterzl, J., and Riha, H., eds., *Developmental Aspects of Antibody Formation and Structure,* Academic Press, New York, p. 485.
Kincade, P. W., Lawton, A. R., Bockman, D. E., and Cooper, M. D., 1970. *Proc. Natl. Acad. Sci.* 67:1918.
Lesley, J., and Dutton , R., 1970. *Science* 169:487.
Marchalonis, J. J., and Nossal, G. J. V., 1968. *Proc. Natl. Acad. Sci.* 61:860.
Mason, S., and Warner, N. L., 1970. *J. Immunol.* 104:762.
McDevitt, H. O., and Benacerraf, B., 1969. *Advan. Immunol.* 11:31.
Miller, J. F. A. P., and Mitchell, G. M., 1969. *Transplant. Rev.* 1:3.
Miller, J. F. A. P., and Sprent, J., 1971. *J. Exptl. Med.* 134:66.
Miller, J. F. A. P., Sprent, J., Basten, A., Warner, N. L., Breitner, J., Rowland, G., Hamilton, J., Silver, H. S., and Martin, W. J., 1971. *J. Exptl. Med.* 134, in press.
Mitchison, N. A., 1967. *Cold Spring Harbor Symp. Quant. Biol.* 32:431.
Mitchison, N. A., Rajewsky, K., and Taylor, R. B., 1970. In Sterzl, J., and Riha, H., eds., *Developmental Aspects of Antibody Formation and Structure,* Academic Press, New York, p. 547.
Naor, D., and Sulitzeanu, D., 1967. *Nature,* 214:687.
Naor, D., and Sulitzeanu, D., 1969. *Internat. Arch. Allergy* 36:112.
Naor, D., Bentwich, Z., and Cividalli, G., 1969. *Aust. J. Exptl. Biol.* 47:759.
Nossal, G. J. V., Warner, N. L., and Lewis, H., 1971. *Cell. Immunol.* 2:41.
Nota, N. R., Liacopoulos Briot, M., Stiffel, C., and Biozzi, G., 1964. *Compt. Rend. Acad. Sci.* 259:1277.
Ovary, Z., and Benacerraf, B., 1963. *Proc. Soc. Exptl. Biol. Med.* 114:72.
Pantelouris, E. M., 1968. *Nature* 217:370.
Pernis, B., Forni, L., and Amante, L., 1970. *J. Exptl. Med.* 132:1001.
Rabellino, E., Colon, S., Grey, H., and Unanue, E., 1970. *J. Exptl. Med.* 133:156.
Raff, M., 1970. *Immunology* 19:637.
Raff, M. C., 1969. *Nature* 224:378.
Raff, M. C., Nase, M., and Mitchison, N. A., 1971. *Nature* 229:50.
Rouse, B. T., and Warner, N. L., 1971. *Cell. Immunol.,* in press.
Rygaard, J., 1969. *Acta Pathol. Microbiol. Scand.* 77:761.
Schlesinger, M., 1970. *Nature* 226:1254.

Sell, S., and Asofsky, R., 1968. *Progr. Allergy* **12**:86.

Sprent, J., and Miller, J. F. A. P., 1971. *Cell. Immunol.,* in press.

Sell, S., Lowe, J. A., and Gell, P. G. H., 1970. *J. Immunol.* **104**:103.

Takahashi, T., Old, L. J., and Boyse, E. A., 1970. *J. Exptl. Med.* **131**:1325.

Thorbecke, G. J., Warner, N. L., Hochwald, G. M., and Ohanian, S. H., 1968. *Immunology* **15**:123.

Till, J. E., and McCulloch, E. A., 1961. *Radiat. Res.* **14**:213.

Tyan, M. L., 1971. *J. Immunol.* **106**:586.

Wang, A. C., Pink, J. R. L., Fudenberg, M. M., and Ohms, J., 1970. *Proc. Natl. Acad. Sci.* **66**:657.

Warner, N. L., 1967. *Folia Biol.* **13**:1.

Warner, N. L., 1971a. Immunogenicity. In Borek, F., ed., *Frontiers in Biology,* North Holland Publishing Co., in press.

Warner, N. L., 1971b. *Transplant. Proc.* **3**:848.

Warner, N. L., and Mason, S., 1971. *Nature,* submitted.

Warner, N. L., Herzenberg, L. A., and Goldstein, G., 1966. *J. Exptl. Med.* **123**:707.

Warner, N. L., Uhr, J. W., Thorbecke, G. J., and Ovary, Z., 1969. *J. Immunol.* **103**:1317.

Warner, N. L., Byrt, P., and Ada, G. L., 1970. *Nature* **226**:942.

Warner, N. L., Ovary, Z., and Kantor, F. S., 1971. *Internat. Arch. Allergy,* in press.

Wigzell, H., and Makela, O., 1970. *J. Exptl. Med.* **132**:110.

Zaalberg, O. B., 1964. *Nature* **202**:123.

Chapter 6

Cellular Basis of Immunological Unresponsiveness

Jacques M. Chiller* and William O. Weigle†
Department of Experimental Pathology
Scripps Clinic and Research Foundation
La Jolla, California

INTRODUCTION

Injection of an antigen into a vertebrate may be followed by a number of different immunological alternatives. Most commonly, a specific immune response is manifested in the form of cell-associated immunity, humoral immunity, or both. In other instances, antigen may specifically prime the challenged host without resulting in expression of a detectable immune response. Finally, antigen may induce the immunological antithesis of a responsive state, that is, a state of specific unresponsiveness. The specific cellular events involved in these differing pathways share at least one facet; i.e., initiation involves the interaction between antigen and a specific cell or cells. The present discussion will consider the experimental data concerning the cellular events and consequences of the interaction between antigen and antigen-reactive cells which lead to the state of specifically induced unresponsiveness. The emphasis will be placed on the cellular phenomena involved in the induction, maintenance, and termination of immunological unresponsiveness as it specifically relates to the block in the formation of humoral antibody.

Publication No. 523 from the Department of Experimental Pathology, Scripps Clinic and Research Foundation. Supported by the United States Public Health Service Grant AI-07007, American Cancer Grant T-519, and Atomic Energy Commission Contract AT(04-3)-410.
* Supported by a Dernham Fellowship (No. J-166) of the California Division of the American Cancer Society.
† Supported by United States Public Health Service Research Career Award 5-K6-GM-6936-10.

119

INDUCTION OF UNRESPONSIVENESS WITH
HETEROLOGOUS SERUM PROTEINS

There are a number of reasons why heterologous serum proteins have been used extensively in studies of induced unresponsiveness. These proteins are soluble and equilibrate rapidly between extra- and intravascular spaces and thus are able to reach all potential antigen-reactive cells. They can be obtained in large quantities and in purified form. They can be trace-labeled with radioactive isotopes and their fate in the host readily followed. Additionally, the immunological reactivity to these antigens can be readily quantitated by sensitive assays which can measure either circulating antibody or antibody-forming cells. As a class of heterologous serum proteins, γ-globulins are endowed with two additional properties favorable for study of the unresponsive state. On one hand, monomeric γ-globulin obtained following ultracentrifugation can induce a complete, specific unresponsive state in adult animals. As will be subsequently described, this state is of relatively long duration (> 100 days) and requires but a single intraperitoneal injection for induction. On the other hand, γ-globulin can be rendered highly immunogenic, without the use of added adjuvants, by heat aggregation. Therefore, two physically distinct forms of the same antigen induce two distinct biological phenomena, namely, responsiveness or unresponsiveness. The monomeric form which induces tolerance will be referred to as a *tolerogen* and its immunological behavior as *tolerogenic*. In contrast, the aggregated form which induces an immune response will be referred to as an *immunogen* and its immunological behavior as *immunogenic*.

Preparations of commercially obtained γ-globulins can be rendered highly tolerogenic if they are made devoid of aggregates by ultracentrifugation (Dresser, 1962). Using human γ-globulin (HGG) as the antigen, this process of deaggregation is extremely reliable for inducing tolerance in mice if attention is paid to other variables. For example, the dose of ultracentrifuged material needed to produce unresponsiveness differs with different strains of mice. C57Bl/6K strain can be made tolerant with 0.1 mg tolerogen, while Balb/cJ mice are not induced to tolerance with as much as 10 mg of tolerogen. Presumably, the difference lies in the efficiency with which these different strains handle trace amounts of aggregated material not removed by the process of ultracentrifugation. More complete deaggregation obtained by Na_2SO_4 salt fractionation produces a monomeric preparation of HGG which is more tolerogenic (Golub and Weigle, 1969). Within a strain, the ease with which unresponsiveness is induced decreases with increased age. Balb/cJ mice can thus be made totally unresponsive to HGG with 5.0 mg of tolerogen at 4 weeks of age but not at 8 weeks of age (von Felten and Weigle, in preparation).

Table I demonstrates the totality and the specificity of an unresponsive

Table I. Induction of Specific Immunological Unresponsiveness to HGG in Adult A/J Mice

Antigen injected		Number of mice	Indirect PFC/10^6 spleen cells	
			Day 30	
Day 0	Days 15 and 25		HGG	TGG
None	0.4 mg AHGG[a]	22	713	ND[b]
2.5 mg DHGG[c]	0.4 mg AHGG	38	0	ND
2.5 mg DHGG	0.4 mg ATGG[d]	10	0	3428

[a]AHGG: aggregated human γ-globulin.

[b]ND: not done.

[c]DHGG: deaggregated human γ-globulin.

[d]ATGG: aggregated turkey γ-globulin.

state induced in adult mice with deaggregated HGG (DHGG). In this case, A/J male mice, 6 weeks of age, were injected intraperitoneally with 2.5 mg DHGG given in a volume of 1.0 ml. The DHGG was obtained by centrifuging DEAE-fractionated HGG (30 mg/ml) at 40,000 rev/min for 150 min in a swinging-bucket rotor. Success in preparing an efficient tolerogen is in part dependent upon careful removal of only the upper third of the centrifuged solution, subsequent dilution to the desired final concentration, and injection into the animal within the shortest time course possible. The data of Table I reveal that mice so treated with tolerogenic HGG are totally unresponsive to subsequent challenges of the immunogenic form of HGG, i.e., heat-aggregated human γ-globulin (AHGG). In contrast, saline-injected controls respond vigorously to such immunogenic challenges. Furthermore, this unresponsive state is specific to HGG, since turkey γ-globulin, an antigen of similar molecular characteristics but antigenically non–cross-reactive with HGG, is able to stimulate a normal response in mice demonstrating total tolerance to HGG. Emphasis should be placed on the fact that the use of a potent immunogen such as AHGG and a sensitive assay of detecting single antibody-forming cells such as the hemolytic plaque system combine to offer this as a most stringent test of a state of specific immunological unresponsiveness and, most important, one which can be quantitated at a cellular level.

KINETICS OF INDUCTION OF IMMUNOLOGICAL
UNRESPONSIVENESS

The exact mechanism by which the state of tolerance is induced is not understood. Alternative viewpoints hold that populations of specifically paralyzed cells exist or that specific clones of cells are killed by the tolerogen or that enhancing antibody masks the immunological potential of otherwise normal cells. In order to offer insight into a possible mechanism, a number of studies have attempted to define the time course for the induction process of unresponsiveness. It would seem likely that a short course of induction would favor a theory encompassing direct interaction between antigen and antigen-reactive cells, since this process would be limited only by the time needed for diffusion or dissemination of tolerogen. On the other hand, a longer induction period would support the contention that some maturational event is a prerequisite for the acquisition of the unresponsive state. Studies concerning kinetics of tolerance induction can be divided according to whether they were performed *in vitro* or *in vivo*.

In Vitro Studies

Diener and Armstrong (1969) found that mouse spleen cells cultured *in vitro* with high concentrations of flagellin from *Salmonella adelaide* were rendered tolerant within a 3 hr period. Similar results are obtained when spleen cells were exposed for various lengths of time to tolerogenic doses of antigen but at a temperature of 4 C instead of 37 C. Similarly, Britton (1969) demonstrated paralysis of normal mouse spleen cells following *in vitro* exposure to high doses of detoxified endotoxin of *Escherichia coli*. In this experiment, exposure for only 2 hr was needed to specifically induce unresponsiveness. Induction of paralysis *in vitro* with heterologous serum proteins has met with limited success. Scott and Waksman (1968) showed that cells obtained from rat lymphoid organs which had been injected *in vitro* with bovine gamma globulin (BGG) were specifically unresponsive when transferred to thymectomized, irradiated hosts. Only a 1 hr incubation period appeared to be necessary for induction. Tolerance to BGG could not be induced following incubation of lymphocyte suspensions with the soluble antigen *in vitro*. The fact that unresponsiveness was obtained when similar suspensions of cells and tolerogen were injected into irradiated hosts suggests that the physiological environment in which antigen and lymphocytes interact is critical and that the milieu of an intact organ or the tissues of an irradiated animal provide the proper setting for optimal interaction between tolerogen and cells. In mice, similar results are obtained with HGG (Sieckman, unpublished). That is, the ease with which unresponsiveness can be induced in adoptively transferred spleen cells with either deaggregated HGG or biologically filtered HGG (Frei et al., 1965) contrasts with the difficulty in achieving this state when the same combination is incubated in vitro.

In Vivo Studies

In contrast to the general agreement on the short time course necessary to induce tolerance in vitro, experiments utilizing in vivo systems have shown varying results as to the duration of the induction process. Thus, using cell transfer experiments, it was found that a period of 5 days was required to induce unresponsiveness in spleen cells of animals treated with high doses of pneumococcal polysaccharides (Matangkasombut and Seastone, 1968), agreeing with the time course previously reported for inducing the unresponsive state with deaggregated HGG (Golub and Weigle, 1967). A similar approach utilized by Mitchison (1968) showed that peripheral blood leukocytes could be rendered unresponsive to high doses of bovine serum albumin (BSA) in 2 hr, whereas spleen cells from similarly treated animals were tolerant only after a 24 hr period. Das and Leskovitz (1970) reported that spleen cells from mice injected with deaggregated bovine γ-globulin (BGG) showed significant unresponsiveness as little as 4 hr after tolerogen treatment. As in the previous experiments, the assay for tolerance was the adoptive transfer of the washed spleen cells into irradiated recipients, which were then immunized and subsequently assayed for the immune elimination of radioactive labeled antigen. Dresser (1969) found that the induction of paralysis in mice to γ-globulin required a longer period of time than that described above. Porcine γ-globulin induced complete tolerance in 4 days and HGG in 15 days, while equine, bovine, rabbit, and chicken γ-globulin required even longer time courses and, in addition, only induced hyporesponsive states.

It is doubtful that the heterogenicity of data on the kinetics of the induction of unresponsiveness presented by these many reports reflects a similar diversity of pathways by which unresponsiveness to heterologous serum proteins is induced. A more likely explanation of these discrepancies may be found in the myriad of differences in the protocols and materials utilized. In addition, limited by the assay systems used in evaluating the immune response, these data fail to provide clear information on the quantitative cellular kinetics of this induction period. Using HGG, quantitation can be readily obtained by assaying for cells forming antibody to HGG using a modification (Golub et al., 1968) of the hemolytic plaque technique (Jerne and Nordin, 1963). Such a cellular quantitation exposes facets of unresponsiveness which may be otherwise inaccessible to serological testing, since extraneous antigen in the circulation could bind to and mask humoral antibody.

This cellular approach was used in the following experiments. Mice were sacrificed at various times after the injection of 2.5 mg of deaggregated HGG, and their spleens were pooled for preparation as a single-cell suspension. A set number of cells was injected intravenously into lethally irradiated syngeneic recipients along with immunogenic HGG (AHGG). Following a second injection of AHGG, the spleens of these irradiated hosts were assayed for the number of HGG-specific plaque-forming cells. In addition, at each time interval, saline-injected controls were used as spleen cell donors in order to ascertain the normal PFC response. At each time interval, the response obtained in the tolerogen-treated group was expressed as a percentage of the response obtained in the saline-treated group, and this percentage was plotted as a function of time following the injection of the tolerogenic material. The entire quantitative kinetic curve shown in Fig. 1 yields the following information about the induction process. In the first 3 hr following tolerogen, no significant degree of unresponsiveness is established. It is likely that this is the time course required for the equilibration of tolerogen between the intra- and extravascular spaces. There occurs a rapid induction of cellular unresponsiveness in the next few hours, so that by 24 hr following administration of tolerogen 85% of the unresponsive state in the spleen appears established. The remaining 15% requires a more prolonged period of time, so that total tolerance is not evident until 120 hr. These data may serve to reconcile the previous conflicting results of the other investigations which attempted to establish a time scale for tolerance induction. Thus, 4-5 days is in fact the

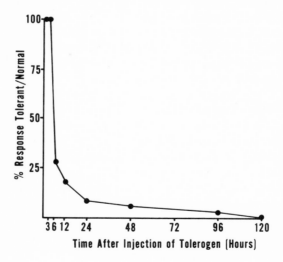

Figure 1. Kinetics of immunological unresponsiveness in the spleens of mice treated with tolerogenic human γ-globulin.

time required for the total establishment of unresponsiveness as described by Golub and Weigle (1967) and Matangkasombut and Seastone (1968) in transfer systems where unresponsiveness was measured qualitatively. However, the fact that unresponsiveness is to a large degree (75%) established by 6 hr after tolerogen injection is also in accord with the *in vivo* reports of Mitchison (1968) and Das and Leskovitz (1970) as well as the *in vitro* studies of Diener and Armstrong (1969) and Britton (1969).

RELATIONSHIP BETWEEN ANTIBODY FORMATION AND THE INDUCTION PROCESS OF UNRESPONSIVENESS

Is the induction of unresponsiveness mediated through an immune mechanism which in the presence of antigen excess leads to a specific clonal exhaustion and subsequent nonreactivity? This view was initially expressed by Sterzl and Trnka (1957) on the basis of data obtained using bacterial antigens. They found that the immune response of newborn rabbits injected with large doses of *Salmonella parathyphi B* was increased and accelerated over that obtained in animals similarly treated with intermediate doses of that antigen. However, when these rabbits as adults were rechallenged with bacteria, their antibody levels were much lower than those of animals primed with lower doses of antigen or of animals not injected with antigens at birth. Similar results were obtained using sheep erythrocytes in newborn piglets and rabbits (Sterzl, 1966). The highest dose of red blood cells given after birth provoked the strongest response in the young of both species. However, following subsequent immunization, the response obtained was lower than that of rabbits injected with lower doses at birth. In light of these results, Sterzl postulated that immunological unresponsiveness resulted from terminal exhaustive differentiation of specifically stimulated cells. Thus, in the presence of excess antigen, the majority of immunologically competent cells differentiated into short-lived antibody-producing cells and therefore were not available to the further injection of specific antigen.

A role for specific antibody in the induction of tolerance to flagellin *in vitro* has been given impetus by the work of Feldmann and Diener (1970). In close analogy to the *in vitro* induction of tolerance using high concentrations of *Salmonella adelaide* H antigens (Diener and Armstrong, 1969), tolerance may also be induced *in vitro* by treating normal mouse spleen cells for 6 hr with low concentrations of the antigen (usually an immunogenic dose) provided that the proper concentration of the specific antibody is also present. Additionally, a cyanogen bromide digest of flagellin (fragment A) which contains all the antigenic determinants that can be recognized on flagellin monomer (Parish and Ada, 1969) and which has no tolerance-inducing capacity at any concentration becomes a potent tolerogen when it is presented to lymphoid cells with specific antibody (Diener and Feldmann, 1970). The authors suggest that immunological tolerance depends on a mechanism which involves the interlinkage of a critical number of antigen receptor sites by antibody. This could be accomplished either by a large number of repeating antigen determinants, as is the case with high doses of polymerized flagellin, or alternatively by the combined action of antigen and antibody, as in the case with low doses of polymerized flagellin and fragment A. Additional support for this theoretical consideration has been provided by Feldmann (1971). Tolerance induction to dinitrophenyl (DNP) in dissociated spleen cell suspensions using dinitrophenyl-polymerized flagellin conjugates was obtained only when these conjugates were highly substituted. Again, the suggestion is made that the induction of unresponsiveness in an antigen-reactive cell involves the simultaneous reaction of many antigenic determinants with the surface of that cell. The need for high DNP density would reflect a requirement that the interaction between cell and determinants occur on a relatively small area of the surface of the cell. The localization of specific receptors on small patchy areas of immunocompetent cells (Mandel et al., 1969) suggests a mechanism by which this requirement can be sterically met.

It remains questionable whether there is universal truth to a hypothesis which demands that a phase of immune activity precede a phase of unresponsiveness. Support or refutation of such a concept might be obtained with adequate testing for antibody formation during the period of induction of immunological tolerance. Since a large amount of antigen is generally required to produce unresponsiveness, the presence or absence of an immune reaction needs to be assessed at a cellular level, where the danger of masking antibody with antigen may be more easily excluded than at the serological level. Utilizing the hemolytic plaque assay for detecting antibody-forming cells, we have investigated this question using three different models of specifically induced unresponsiveness: (1) unresponsiveness induced in adult mice using deaggregated HGG, (2) unresponsiveness induced in newborn rabbits using BSA and, (3) unresponsiveness induced in adult rabbits using large repetitive doses of BSA.

ADULT MICE RENDERED UNRESPONSIVE TO HGG

Mice were injected either with a tolerogenic dose of deaggregated HGG or with an immunogenic challenge of aggregated HGG. At various times after the antigen injections, groups of tolerogen-treated and immunogen-treated mice were sacrificed and their individual spleens assayed for PFC to HGG. As can be seen in Table II, there is an absence of antibody-forming cells as long

Table II. The Immune Response of A/J Mice Injected with Either Aggregated or Deaggregated HGG as Measured by the Presence of Antibody-Forming Cells (PFC) in the Spleen

Day after injection	Indirect PFC/10^6 spleen cells[a]	
	Deaggregated HGG	Aggregated HGG
1	0	0
2	0	0
3	0	5
4	0	26
5	0	64
6	0	91
7	0	105
8	0	53
10	0	18
13	0	5
19	0	7

[a] Ten animals for each group.

as 19 days following exposure to the tolerogenic form of the antigen. In contrast, mice injected with immunogen are seen to contain antibody-forming cells as early as 3 days following challenge. Therefore, within the limits of the sensitivity of the present assay, the induction of unresponsiveness to HGG in adult mice is not accompanied by a phase of antibody formation.

NEWBORN RABBITS RENDERED UNRESPONSIVE TO BSA

Immunological unresponsiveness was induced in rabbits by two subcutaneous injections of 150 mg and 250 mg soluble bovine serum albumin given on the first and third days of life, respectively. At various times, spleens, thymuses, and appendixes of these animals were assayed for the presence of antibody-forming cells specific to BSA. None were detected in any of the organs tested for as long as 19 days following the second neonatal injection (Fig. 2). The failure to find PFC to BSA was specific, since the injection in the same animal of soluble BSA and either aggregated HGG or HGG incorporated into complete Freund's adjuvant stimulated the appearance of PFC to HGG but none to BSA. It should be noted that neonatal rabbits have the capacity to respond to BSA if that antigen is presented in the proper form.

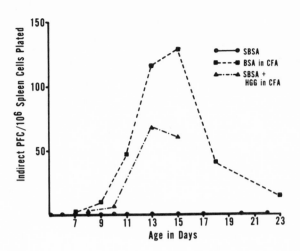

Figure 2. Quantitation of antibody-forming cells (PFC) to either bovine serum albumin (BSA) or human γ-globulin (HGG) in spleens of neonatal rabbits. Spleens were assayed at various times following the injection of either 500 mg soluble BSA or 500 mg soluble BSA and 2 mg HGG in complete Freund's adjuvant (CFA) or 2 mg HGG in CFA alone.

Thus, injecting rabbits on the day of birth with BSA incorporated into complete Freund's adjuvant yields specific antibody-forming cells as early as 10 days later and shows a peak response (day 15) comparable to the response observed in adult rabbits. Therefore, in this second model of unresponsiveness, there is again the lack of antibody formation detectable in the induction process of tolerance.

ADULT RABBITS RENDERED UNRESPONSIVE TO BSA

It was originally shown by Dixon and Maurer (1955) that daily injection of large doses of BSA into adult rabbits produces a state of specific immuno-logical paralysis. Under such condition, it would be predictably impossible to assess serologically the existence of a simultaneous state of immunological reactivity, since the presence of large amounts of antigen in the circulation would be expected to neutralize serum antibody. But, in fact, animals treated with such large doses of antigen do possess antibody-forming cells, as shown in the following experiment. Adult rabbits were injected daily with 1 g of

soluble BSA. At various time intervals, groups of animals were evaluated for
the number of antibody-forming cells to BSA in their spleens. Figure 3 reveals
that there exists in these animals a transient period during which PFC can be
detected. The pattern of this response is similar in time and in magnitude to
that observed in normal rabbits given a single intravenous injection of 20 mg
of BSA. However, whereas the latter group would respond anamnestically to a
secondary challenge of the same antigen, the animals given the course of
repetitive large doses of BSA are unable to demonstrate PFC in response to
this continued injection of antigen. Several additional facets of this experiment should be emphasized. First, unresponsiveness produced in this manner
is of long duration. Although the course of antigen injection was terminated
at day 36, no evidence of antibody-forming cells could be found as long as 93
days following the initial day of injection. Second, unresponsiveness is specific. Animals injected at day 8 or at day 30 with human γ-globulin while
undergoing the paralytic treatment with BSA in both instances could respond
to HGG. Third, unresponsiveness is demonstrable even with the use of a
highly immunogenic form of BSA. That is, animals challenged on day 29 with
BSA incorporated into complete Freund's adjuvant produced no splenic PFC
to BSA. Fourth, the lack of antibody in the circulation of unresponsive animals does not mean a similar lack of antibody-producing cells. Thus, at no

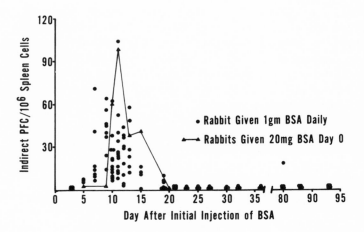

Figure 3. Cellular response (PFC) of rabbits following a paralytic
course of bovine serum albumin (BSA). Rabbits were injected with
daily subcutaneous injections of 1 g BSA for 36 days. Each point on
the graph represents the PFC to BSA in the spleen of an individual
rabbit so treated. The solid line represents the cellular response of a
group of rabbits given a single intravenous injection of 20 mg BSA.

time during the time course of the experiment was there demonstrable circulating antibody to BSA, even though PFC were present in high number in the spleens of the same animals.

Immunological paralysis to pneumococcal polysaccharides may also be the product of divergent mechanisms. Howard *et al.* (1970) demonstrated that following the injection of 2-50 μg SIII antigen, mice have little or no hemagglutinating antibody in the circulation, but their spleens contain a great number of PFC to the pneumococcal polysaccharide. This apparent state of unresponsiveness is interpreted by the authors to reflect "pseudoparalysis," where antigen masks peripherally the intensity of a cellular immune response. However, animals receiving 50 μg or more SIII display neither circulating antibody nor splenic antibody-forming cells. This is viewed as true paralysis, since the lack of peripheral antibody is due to a central inhibition of the immune system. It is interesting that this group of investigators had previously reported that the spleens of mice rendered tolerant with 500 μg SIII contained a considerable number of rosette-forming cells (RFC) to the antigen—in fact, greater numbers than were seen in optimally immunized animals (Howard *et al.*, 1969). The presence of RFC and a concomitant absence of PFC in mice tolerant to detoxified *E. coli* lipopolysaccharide have also been reported by Sjöberg (1971). He concludes that tolerance to polysaccharides is the specific inhibition of the process which leads to the development of antibody-forming cells without simultaneously affecting the process leading to the development of antigen-binding cells or RFC. It may well be that in the unresponsive states which were studied in which no evidence for PFC during the induction process could be found (Chiller and Weigle, 1971; Chiller *et al.*, 1971a), there could exist an increase in RFC specific to the tolerated antigens. Before engaging in such a search, technical modifications of the rosette test should be made so as to totally eliminate the background RFC which plague this assay. Otherwise, it is difficult to be confident of the biological significance of a minute increase above that background number.

Binding of highly radioactive labeled antigen to specific lymphocytes can be visualized technically by means of radioautography using either light or electron microscopy. The first to explore and to verify the feasibility of such an approach were Naor and Sulitzeanu (1967), and their findings were subsequently extended independently by Ada (1970) and by Humphrey and Keller (1970). It would appear that the antigen-binding reaction assay might be a way by which to test the concepts of cell inactivation *vs.* cell deletion as means of achieving the unresponsive state. The data so far reported have given ambiguous answers. Naor and Sulitzeanu (1969) concluded that compared to normal mice, mice tolerant to BSA showed a reduced number of cells binding the labeled antigen. Humphrey and Keller (1970) examined spleens and lymph nodes of mice made tolerant either to hemocyanin or to the synthetic multichain polypeptide TGAL [(T,G)-A-L]. Little reduction of total antigen-binding cells was found, compared to the number visible in nontreated animals. There appeared to be a significant reduction of the number of the most heavily labeled cells in tolerant animals, but only small numbers were examined. Ada (1970) was unable to find significant differences between the numbers of cells reacting with antigens in either normal or unresponsive rats. Two separate antigens were used, and with each (flagellin and hemocyanin) the frequency of binding cells categorized according to intensity of labeling was similar for the spleens of normal and tolerant animals. The data obtained by this elegant experimental approach should be viewed with some reservation. What proportion of the antigen-binding cells which exist in nonimmunized animals is relevant to the immune process which follows interaction between antigen and cell? If this percentage were small, then the noise provided by the irrelevant cells could be expected to conceal a deletion process in an unresponsive state. Obviously, the biological conclusions which can be obtained from this technique require a correlation between cells binding radioactive antigens and cells participating in an immunological reaction.

In summary, it appears that the demonstration of a stage of immunity during the onset of immunological unresponsiveness is largely dependent on the states of unresponsiveness studied and the conditions with which they are induced. These results emphasize that unresponsiveness should be treated as merely the final product of experimental manipulations. Depending on the conditions utilized, the end results may well be identical—i.e., specific unresponsiveness—but the mechanism by which they are achieved may involve alternative pathways. For this reason, a single unique scheme by which tolerance is induced may prove to be elusive.

CELLULAR SITES OF IMMUNOLOGICAL UNRESPONSIVENESS

An evaluation of the specific cellular lesion of immune unresponsiveness demands knowledge of which cells participate in evoking immune responsiveness. There is increased awareness of the complexity of the cellular events involved in the initiation of the primary immune response. This has been provided in part by discovery of several participating cell types, so that macrophages, lymphoid cells derived from thymus, and lymphoid cells derived from bone marrow may all collaborate in the response to certain antigens.

Macrophages

A requirement for macrophage-like cells for the initiation of a primary response to sheep erythrocytes was first detailed by Mosier (1967). Using the *in vitro* technique developed by Mishell and Dutton (1967), he found that a mouse spleen cell preparation could be physically subdivided into cells which were adherent to plastic and those which were nonadherent. Neither of these populations alone could be induced to form antibody to the heterologous red blood cells but would do so when they were recombined.

The exact role which macrophages play in immune responses is not really clear. There exists evidence that they process antigens in a manner so as to increase their immunogenicity, perhaps by concentrating and retaining immunogenic molecules on their plasma membranes. For example, hemocyanin extracted from *Maia spinado* is 30-40 times more effective in priming mice when it is bound to macrophages than is its soluble form (Unanue and Askonas, 1968). However, this enhanced immunogenicity is greatly reduced if the macrophages are either trypsinized or treated with specific antibody, suggesting that surface-bound antigen has either been removed or covered (Unanue and Cerottini, 1970). Similarly, bovine and human serum albumins are rendered more highly immunogenic following uptake by macrophages (Mitchison, 1969*a*).

Whatever part may be played by macrophages, there is little doubt that it is one which is immunologically nonspecific, since macrophages from tolerant animals are capable of handling the antigen to which the animal is tolerant in the same way as cells from normal animals. This was observed by Harris (1967), who reported that peritoneal cells from normal rabbits or rabbits tolerant to BGG took up the antigen and specifically stimulated the rate of DNA synthesis in spleen cell suspensions from immunized rabbits to the same extent. Similarly, Mitchison (1969*a*) concluded that a similar response is evoked whether peritoneal cells are obtained from normal mice or mice unresponsive to BSA.

Thymus-Derived and Bone Marrow-Derived Cells

There now exist ample data to support the concept that parts of the immune response to certain antigens are played by cells derived from the thymus in cooperation with cells derived from the bone marrow (Claman and Chaperon, 1969; Miller and Mitchell, 1969; Taylor, 1969). Although all lymphoid stem cells originate from the bone marrow, those which reside for part of their life in the thymus have been called *thymus-dependent, thymus-derived,* or *T cells.* Those which pass directly from bone marrow to peripheral lymphoid tissues are called *bone marrow-derived* or *B cells*, perhaps analogous to cells derived from the bursa of Fabricius of birds.

Evidence for the direct cooperation between T lymphocytes and B lymphocytes was provided initially by the observation of Claman *et al.* (1966), who showed that the γM hemolysin response to sheep erythrocytes of lethally irradiated mice was far greater when both thymus and bone marrow cells were used for reconstitution of the host than the sum of the responses obtained when each cell type was injected alone. This observation has been confirmed using other antigens such as heterologous serum proteins (Taylor, 1969; Habicht et al., 1970), and cooperation appears to be the cellular basis for the hapten-carrier system in immunity (Mitchison et al., 1970).

The precise way in which these cells cooperate is not clear. From the observations by Mitchell and Miller (1968), it is known that it is the bone marrow-derived cell which actually synthesizes antibody. It has been suggested by Mitchison (1969b) that the thymus cell acts by binding antigen on its surface so as to provide a higher concentration of localized antigen for stimulation of B cells than if the antigen were simply dispersed throughout the body. Alternatively, the suggestion has been put forth that a mitogenic factor is released by specifically stimulated T cells which is required for the proliferation of specifically stimulated B cells (Dutton, 1971). It is probable that the helper role played by thymus cells will turn out to be one which lowers the effective concentration of antigen needed to stimulate an immune response by B lymphocytes. In accordance with the latter concept, high doses of antigens appear to obviate the requirement for thymus cells seen with low doses (Sinclair and Elliott, 1968), and certain antigens which have repeated antigenic determinants (polysaccharides) are not dependent on thymocytes for their immunogenicity (Möller, 1970).

There have been a number of studies which have been concerned with the determination of the capacity of B and T cells to be rendered immunologically unresponsive. It is generally agreed that thymus cells or their derivatives can be made tolerant. This conclusion was reached initially by Isakovic et al. (1965), who showed that although normal thymus grafts were able to restore responsiveness to thymectomized, irradiated, bone marrow-protected mice, thymus grafts from specifically tolerant animals could not. Taylor (1969) found that lethally irradiated mice given normal bone marrow and thymus cells obtained from donor mice pretreated with 10 mg BSA 24 hr before sacrifice were unable to respond to BSA. Many and Schwartz (1970) found that thymocytes from mice made tolerant following treatment with sheep erythrocytes and cyclophosphamide specifically failed to act synergistically with normal bone marrow cells. Using the same manner of inducing tolerance, Miller and Mitchell (1970) reported that only peripheralized thymocytes such as those found in the thoracic duct lymph could be rendered unresponsive. With respect to cyclophosphamide-induced tolerance, it is assumed that the drug specifically affects those cells which are induced to differentiate or proliferate following specific interaction with antigen. Since the T-cell population appears to be the one initially stimulated by antigen (Davies et al., 1966), it is to be the expected site of the lesion in cyclophosphamide-induced tolerance. Inasmuch as the basis of cellular cooperation appears to lie in the helper effect of T cells on the stimulation of B cells, any event which leads to specific T-cell suicide must concomitantly leave an unstimulated B-cell population, free, therefore, from the effects of cyclophosphamide.

Evidence for specific tolerance in bone marrow is not nearly as prevalent in the literature. Playfair (1969) reported that tolerance to erythrocytes can be found to exist in the marrow of (NZB $\times$ Balb/C)F_1 mice, an observation more recently confirmed by Talal (1971). Gershon and Kondo (1970) demonstrated that tolerance could be induced with large doses of sheep erythrocytes for a short period of time and that this state of unresponsiveness was dependent on the presence of tolerant thymus cells. Our own approach to the problem was predicated on the notion that the investigation of thymus cell and bone marrow cell tolerance demanded a system in which a total state of unresponsiveness could be specifically induced without the requirement for either drugs or repeated large challenges. As described above, human γ-globulin unresponsiveness in adult mice provides such a system.

Following the demonstration that cellular collaboration between thymus and bone marrow occurred in the response to HGG (Habicht et al., 1970), it was shown that both of these cell types could be rendered specifically unresponsive with the tolerogen (Chiller et al., 1970). In these experiments mice were injected with deaggregated HGG, and 17 days later the animals were sacrificed and single-cell preparations of their thymus or bone marrow were injected along with normal bone marrow or thymus cells, respectively, into lethally irradiated syngeneic recipients. At the same time, the animals were challenged with both aggregated human and turkey γ-globulins. After a second challenge with these two immunogens, spleens from these mice were assessed for the number of plaque-forming cells specific to HGG or TGG. As can be seen in Table III, a response to HGG was evident only when both thymus and bone marrow cells came from normal donor mice. The failure of either thymus cells or bone marrow cells to collaborate in the response to HGG was specific, since all cell combinations tested responded in a normal fashion to the non-cross-reacting antigen TGG. This established that specificity lies both at thymus and at bone marrow levels and predicted that unresponsiveness in a single cell type would be sufficient to make an intact animal appear unresponsive. That such a state of cellular dichotomy does exist was demonstrated in the following experiment (Chiller et al., 1971b). The kinetic pattern for the induction, maintenance, and spontaneous loss of tolerance to deaggregated HGG was determined in thymus cells, in bone marrow cells, and in the whole animal. Experimentally, the protocol followed was essentially that described before with the exception that thymus cells and bone marrow cells were obtained from animals at various time intervals following their treatment with

Table III.   Specificity of Unresponsiveness in Thymus Cells and Bone Marrow
Cells Obtained from Mice Previously Injected with Tolerogenic HGG[a]

Cell combinations	Indirect PFC/spleen to	
	TGG	HGG
nT + nBM	9,824	2508
tT + nBM	23,296	0
nt + tBM	22,425	0
tT + tBM	9,797	0

[a] n, cells from normal donors; t, cells from tolerogen-treated donors; T, thymus; BM, bone
marrow; TGG, turkey γ-globulin; HGG, human γ-globulin.

tolerogen. At each interval of time, the response obtained in the recipients
receiving one cell type from tolerogen-treated donors and one cell type obtained from noninjected donors, compared to the response obtained in the
recipients of both normal cell types, was expressed as a degree of unresponsiveness and plotted as shown in Fig. 4. Several interesting observations can be
made. The kinetic pattern for each cell population is distinct. Bone marrow
cells do not begin to show unresponsiveness until after 8 days following the
injection of tolerogen. Total unresponsiveness in these cells is not achieved
until later, around day 21. By day 49, however, tolerance in bone marrow

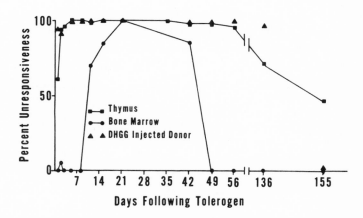

Figure 4.   Kinetics of immunological unresponsiveness in mice, their
thymus cells, and their bone marrow cells following injection of deaggregated human γ-globulin.

cells has spontaneously terminated, and bone marrow cells from such an animal can respond as well as cells from a normal mouse. In contrast, thymus cells are rendered unresponsive much faster and maintain this state for a much longer period of time before they, too, spontaneously return to normality between days 135 and 150. The whole animal behaves with a kinetic pattern essentially superimposable on that described for thymus cells. It can be concluded from these results that an animal may appear tolerant and yet be a cellular composite of two cell populations with differing immunological potential, that is, unresponsive T lymphocytes and normal B lymphocytes.

In addition to a difference in their distinct kinetic pattern of unresponsiveness, bone marrow and thymus cells also differ in their sensitivity to varying doses of tolerogen. It can be seen in Table IV that the injection of 2.5, 0.5, 0.1, and 0.01 mg of deaggregated HGG induces tolerance in thymus cells, whereas bone marrow cells are affected only with 2.5 and 0.5 mg of tolerogen and even then not completely. No evidence for the induction of unresponsiveness at either cellular level was obtained at extremely low doses of tolerogen (10^{-11} or 10^{-13} mg).

In summary, both thymus cells and bone marrow cells can be made tolerant to HGG. Bone marrow cells require higher doses of tolerogen for the induction of specific unresponsiveness, they require a longer induction period, and in these cells the unresponsive state is of shorter duration than in thymus cells. These findings now allow speculation on the cellular basis and dynamics involved in previously described phenomena of immunology for which a cellular interpretation has been lacking. One which presently will be considered in detail is the induced termination of tolerance.

Table IV. Effect of Dose of Tolerogen (Deaggregated HGG) on the Induction of Unresponsiveness in Thymus Cells and Bone Marrow Cells of Adult A/J Mice[a]

Dose of tolerogen injected (mg)	Percent unresponsiveness in	
	Thymus	Bone marrow
2.5	99	70
0.5	99	56
0.1	94	9
0.01	54	0
10^{-11}	0	0
10^{-13}	0	0

[a] Eleven days after the injection of tolerogen.

TERMINATION OF IMMUNOLOGICAL UNRESPONSIVENESS

The induced state of specific unresponsiveness will either terminate spontaneously, as indicated above, or can be actively terminated by the injection of certain cross-reactive antigens (Weigle, 1961) or preparations of the tolerated antigen which have been appropriately altered (Weigle, 1962). Rabbits made tolerant by neonatal injections of 500 mg BSA make antibody reactive with BSA if as adults (3 months of age) they are challenged with cross-reacting albumins. It is important that the degree of cross-reactivity not be too close. Thus, albumins from pig, human, horse, and guinea pig which cross react with BSA 30, 15, 15, and 6%, respectively, all terminate the unresponsive state, while sheep serum albumin which cross-reacts 75% with BSA usually fails to elicit an immune response in these tolerant animals (Weigle, 1964). Recent data indicate that normal rabbits and rabbits tolerant to BSA make similar amounts of both precipitating and binding antibody to that antigen following immunization with aqueous preparations of any one of the four cross-reacting albumins (Benjamin and Weigle, 1970). The avidity of the antibody so produced is dependent solely on the antigen used to terminate the unresponsive state and not on whether the antibody is made by normal or unresponsive animals. Thus, following injection of normal and unresponsive rabbits with cross-reacting heterologous albumins, no quantitative or qualitative difference in the anti-BSA response can be detected. An analogous case can be made for the termination of natural tolerance to thyroglobulin (Weigle, 1965). These data strongly suggest that tolerant animals may possess the full potential to produce antibody specific to the tolerated antigen but lack the ability to recognize the antigen as an immunogenic molecule, so that these cells cannot be turned on to the synthesis of specific antibody. The data on the collaboration of two cell types in the induction of an immune response provide a clue to these observations if thymus cells recognize the immunogenic cross-reacting molecule and bone marrow cells are responsive to the tolerated antigen and produce antibody. If the results obtained with HGG in the mouse system can be extrapolated to the data obtained in rabbits with BSA, rabbits in which unresponsiveness to this heterologous serum albumin had been induced at birth would be expected to contain at the time of testing (90 days after treatment with tolerogen) thymus cells which are unresponsive but bone marrow cells that have recovered from the unresponsive state. However, these animals would possess thymus cells with specificity toward the cross-reacting antigens. Therefore, collaboration between these thymus cells (via determinants specific to the terminating antigen) and the bone marrow cells (via determinants cross-reacting with the tolerated antigen) could lead to a normal response to such cross-reacting determinants. The stimulation of bone marrow cells in this manner would result in their proliferation, differentiation, and subsequent synthesis of antibody with a specificity analogous to the receptor sites on those cells.

In the case of termination of tolerance to thyroglobulins, the known low levels of circulating protein (Daniels *et al.*, 1967) would, in a situation analogous to the dose response to tolerogenic HGG in the mouse system, be sufficient to render only thymus cells unresponsive but not bone marrow cells. Accordingly, cross-reacting thyroglobulins could be recognized as immunogenic by thymus cells and stimulate bone marrow cells to synthesize antibody specific for native thyroglobulin. This hypothesis gains support from the observation that thymus and bone marrow cells may each react with different determinants on an antigen molecule (Mitchison *et al.*, 1970).

The induction of unresponsiveness to a given antigen usually incapacitates the entire spectrum of immune reactivity. It was observed that tolerance to picryl chloride spans not only contact dermatitis due to delayed hypersensitivity but also the formation of both γ_1 and γ_2 circulating antibody (Chase, 1963). The same appears true for tolerance to heterologous proteins, since in guinea pigs rendered tolerant to BSA or HGG, both circulating antibody and delayed hypersensitivity are suppressed (Humphrey and Turk, 1961). However, a number of cases have been reported which demonstrate only partial tolerance of the immune system. It is interesting that all such reports show a common selective suppression of delayed hypersensitivity without a concomitant effect on the production of humoral antibody. For example, Turk and Humphrey (1961) showed that guinea pigs made tolerant to HGG were subsequently able to respond by making circulating antibody against this protein but did not display delayed hypersensitivity toward the antigen. Borel *et al.* (1966) suppressed specifically delayed hypersensitivity but not formation of circulating antibody as a result of injecting newborn guinea pigs with DNP-BGG. Battisto and Chase (1965) were able to stimulate the formation of antibodies by immunization with hapten-carrier conjugates in animals rendered tolerant by oral administration of the antigen. However, the animals remained nonreactive for delayed hypersensitivity. Crowle and Hsu (1966) showed similarly that in mice delayed hypersensitivity can be preferentially suppressed. Finally, Bast *et al.* (1971) have also found this dissociation between delayed hypersensitivity and antibody formation in guinea pigs recovering from a state of tolerance to HSA.

These examples have occurred too frequently to be dismissed simply as fortuitous. In view of the cellular dynamics involved in unresponsiveness, it is tempting to interpret these findings as selective unresponsiveness in T cells without concomitant tolerance in B cells. Implicit in this consideration is the assumption that T lymphocytes after stimulation with specific antigen are able to mediate reactions of delayed hypersensitivity and/or cooperate with B lymphocytes in the production of humoral antibody. Their specific inactivation would eliminate states of delayed hypersensitivity, while B lymphocytes, potentially able to respond to antigen stimulation, might do so under conditions of alternative helper mechanisms or with extensive immunological challenge.

REFERENCES

Ada, G. L., 1970. Antigen binding cells in tolerance and immunity. *Transplant. Rev.* 5:105.

Bast, R. C., Jr., Manseau, E. G., and Dvorak, H. F., 1971. Heterogenicity of the cellular immune response. I. Kinetics of lymphocyte stimulation during sensitization and recovery from tolerance. *J. Exptl. Med.* 133:187.

Battisto, J. R., and Chase, M. W., 1965. Induced unresponsiveness to simple allergenic chemicals. II. Independence of delayed-type hypersensitivity and formation of circulating antibody. *J. Exptl. Med.* 121:591.

Benjamin, D. C., and Weigle, W. O., 1970. The termination of immunological unresponsiveness to bovine serum albumin in rabbits. I. Quantitative and qualitative response to cross-reacting albumins. *J. Exptl. Med.* 132:66.

Borel, Y., Fairconnet, M., and Miescher, P. A., 1966. Selective suppression of delayed hypersensitivity by the induction of immunologic tolerance. *J. Exptl. Med.* 123:585.

Britton, S., 1969. Regulation of antibody synthesis against *Escherichia coli* endotoxin. IV. Induction of paralysis in vitro by treating normal lymphoid cells with antigen. *J. Exptl. Med.* 129:469.

Chase, M. W., 1963. In *Tolerance acquise et le tolerance naturelle a l'egard de substances antigeniques definies,* Centre National de le Reserche Scientifique, Paris, p. 139.

Chiller, J. M., and Weigle, W. O., 1971. Cellular events during the induction of immunologic unresponsiveness in adult mice. *J. Immunol.,* 106:1647.

Chiller, J. M., Habicht, G. S., and Weigle, W. O., 1970. Cellular sites of immunologic unresponsiveness. *Proc. Natl. Acad. Sci.* 65:551.

Chiller, J. M., Habicht, G. S., and Weigle, W. O., 1971a. Kinetic differences in unresponsiveness of thymus and bone marrow cells. *Science* 171:813.

Chiller, J. M., Romball, C., and Weigle, W. O., 1971b. Induction of immunologic unresponsiveness in neonatal and adult rabbits. Difference in the cellular events. *J. Exptl. Med.*

Claman, H. N., and Chaperon, E. A., 1969. Immunologic complementation between thymus and bone marrow cells. A model for the two-cell theory of immunocompetence. *Transplant. Rev.* 1:92.

Claman, H. N., Chaperon, E. A., and Triplett, R. F., 1966. Thymus–marrow cell combinations. Synergism in antibody production. *Proc. Soc. Exptl. Biol. Med.* 122:1167.

Crowle, A. J., and Hsu, C. C., 1966. Split tolerance affecting delayed hypersensitivity and induced in mice by pre-immunization with protein antigens in solution. *Clin. Exptl. Immunol.* 1:323.

Daniels, P. M., Pratt, O. E., Roitt, I. M., and Torrigiani, G., 1967. The release of thyroglobulin from the thyroid gland into thyroid lymphatics; the identification of thyroglobulin in the thyroid lymph and in the blood of monkeys by physical and immunological methods and its estimation by radioimmunoassay. *Immunology* 12:489.

Das, S., and Leskovitz, S., 1970. The kinetics of in vivo tolerance induction in mice. *J. Immunol.* 106:438.

Davies, A. J. S., Leuchars, E., Wallis, V., and Koller, P. C., 1966. The mitotic response of thymus-derived cells to antigenic stimulus. *Transplantation* 4:438.

Diener, E., and Armstrong, W. D., 1969. Immunological tolerance in vitro. Kinetic studies at the cellular level. *J. Exptl. Med.* **129**:591.

Diener, E., and Feldmann, M., 1970. Antibody mediated suppression of the immune response in vitro. II. A new approach to the phenomenon of immunologic tolerance. *J. Exptl. Med.* **132**:31.

Dixon, F. J., and Maurer, P. H., 1955. Immunologic unresponsiveness induced by protein antigens. *J. Exptl. Med.* **101**:245.

Dresser, D. W., 1962. Specific inhibition of antibody production. II. Paralysis induced in adult mice by small quantities of protein antigens. *Immunology* **5**:378.

Dresser, D. W., 1969. The rates of induction and loss of immunological paralysis. *Internat. Arch. Allergy.* **35**:253.

Dutton, R. W., 1971. In Amos, B., ed., *Progress in Immunology,* Academic Press, New York, in press.

Feldmann, M., 1971. Induction of immunity and tolerance to the dinitrophenyl determinant in vitro. *Nature, New Biol.* **231**:21.

Feldmann, M., and Diener, E., 1970. Antibody mediated suppression of the immune response in vitro. I. Evidence for a central effect. *J. Exptl. Med.* **131**:247.

Frei, P. C., Benacerraf, B., and Thorbecke, G. J., 1965. Phagocytosis of the antigen, a crucial step in the induction of the primary response. *Proc. Natl. Acad. Sci.* **53**:20.

Gershon, R. K., and Kondo, K., 1970. Cell interaction in the induction of tolerance. The role of thymic lymphocytes. *Immunology* **18**:721.

Golub, E. S., and Weigle, W. O., 1967. Studies on the induction of immunologic unresponsiveness. II. Kinetics. *J. Immunol.* **99**:624.

Golub, E. S., and Weigle, W. O., 1969. Studies on the induction of immunologic unresponsiveness. III. Antigen form and mouse strain variation. *J. Immunol.* **102**:389.

Golub, E. S., Mishell, R. I., Weigle, W. O., and Dutton, R. W., 1968. A modification of the hemolytic plaque assay for use with protein antigens. *J. Immunol.* **100**:133.

Habicht, G. S., Chiller, J. M., and Weigle, W. O., 1970. Absence of plaque-forming cells in animals immunologically unresponsive to protein antigens. In Sterzl, J., and Riha, I., eds., *Developmental Aspects of Antibody Formation and Structure,* Academia, Prague, p. 893.

Harris, G., 1967. Macrophages from tolerant rabbits as mediators of a specific immunological response in vitro. *Immunology* **12**:159.

Howard, J. G., Elson, J., Christie, G. H., and Kinsky, R. G., 1969. Studies on immunological paralysis. II. The detection and significance of antibody-forming cells in the spleen during immunological paralysis with type III pneumococcal polysaccharide. *Clin. Exptl. Immunol.* **4**:41.

Howard, J. G., Christie, G. H., and Courtenay, B. M., 1970. Treadmill neutralization of antibody and central inhibition. Separate components of pneumococcal polysaccharide paralysis. *Transplantation* **10**:351.

Humphrey, J. H., and Keller, H. U., 1970. Some evidence for specific interaction between immunologically competent cells and antigens. In Sterzl, J., and Riha, I., eds., *Developmental Aspects of Antibody Formation and Structure,* Academia, Prague, p. 485.

Humphrey, J. H., and Turk, J. L., 1961. Immunological unresponsiveness in guinea pigs. I. Immunological unresponsiveness to heterologous serum proteins. *Immunology* **4**:301.

Isakovic, K., Smith, S. B., and Waksman, B. H., 1965. Role of the thymus in tolerance. I. Tolerance to bovine gamma globulin in thymectomized, irradiated rats grafted with thymus from tolerant donors. *J. Exptl. Med.* **122**:1103.

Jerne, N. K., and Nordin, A. A., 1963. Plaque formation in agar by single antibody producing cells. *Science* **140**:405.

Mandel, T., Byrt, P., and Ada, G. L., 1969. Morphological examination of antigen reactive cells in the mouse spleen and peritoneal cavity. *Exptl. Cell Res.* **58**:179.

Many, A., and Schwartz, R. S., 1970. Drug induced immunologic tolerance: Site of action of cyclophosphamide. *Proc. Soc. Exptl. Biol. Med.* **133**:754.

Matangkasombut, P., and Seastone, C. V., 1968. Sequence of events in mice early in immunologic paralysis by pneumococcal polysaccharide. *J. Immunol.* **100**:845.

Miller, J. F. A. P., and Mitchell, G. F., 1969. Thymus and antigen-reactive cells. *Transplant. Rev.* **1**:3.

Miller, J. F. A. P., and Mitchell, G. F., 1970. Cell to cell interaction in the immune response. V. Target cells for tolerance induction. *J. Exptl. Med.* **131**:675.

Mishell, R. I., and Dutton, R. W., 1967. Immunization of dissociated spleen cell cultures from normal mice. *J. Exptl. Med.* **126**:423.

Mitchell, G. F., and Miller, J. F. A. P., 1968. Cell to cell interaction in the immune response. II. The source of hemolysin-forming cells in irradiated mice given bone marrow and thymus or thoracic duct lymphocytes. *J. Exptl. Med.* **128**:821.

Mitchison, N. A., 1968. Immunological paralysis induced by brief exposure of cells to protein antigens. *Immunology* **15**:531.

Mitchison, N. A., 1969a. The immunogenic capacity of antigen taken up by peritoneal exudates. *Immunology* **16**:1.

Mitchison, N. A., 1969b. Immunocompetent cell populations. In Landy, M., and Braun, W., eds., *Immunological Tolerance,* Academic Press, New York, p. 115.

Mitchison, N. A., Rajewsky, K., and Taylor, R. B., 1970. Cooperation of antigenic determinants and of cells in the induction of antibodies. In Sterzl, J., and Riha, I., eds., *Developmental Aspects of Antibody Formation and Structure,* Academia, Prague, p. 547.

Möller, G., 1970. Immunocyte triggering. *Cell Immunol.* **1**:573.

Mosier, D. E., 1967. A requirement for two cell types for antibody formation in vitro. *Science* **158**:1575.

Naor, D., and Sulitzeanu, D., 1967. Binding of radioactive bovine serum albumin to mouse spleen cells. *Nature* **214**:687.

Naor, D., and Sulitzeanu, D., 1969. Binding of I^{125}-BSA to lymphoid cells of tolerant mice. *Internat. Arch. Allergy* **36**:112.

Parish, C. R., and Ada, G. L., 1969. The tolerance inducing properties in rats of bacterial flagellin cleaved at the methionine residues. *Immunology* **17**:153.

Playfair, J. H. L., 1969. Specific tolerance to sheep erythrocytes in mouse bone marrow cells. *Nature* **222**:882.

Scott, D. W., and Waksman, B. H., 1968. Tolerance in vitro: Suppression of immune responsiveness to bovine γ-globulin after injection of antigen into intact lymphoid organs. *J. Immunol.* **100**:912.

Sinclair, N. R. St. C., and Elliott, E. V., 1968. Neonatal thymectomy and the decrease in antigen sensitivity of the primary response and immunological "memory" systems. *Immunology* **15**:325.

Sjöberg, O., 1971. Antigen-binding cells in mice immune or tolerant to *Escherichia coli* polysaccharides. *J. Exptl. Med.* **133**:1015.

Sterzl, J., 1966. Immunological tolerance as the result of terminal differentiation of immunologically competent cells. *Nature* **209**:416.

Sterzl, J., and Trnka, Z., 1957. Effect of very large doses of bacterial antigen on antibody production in newborn rabbits. *Nature* **179**:918.

Talal, N., 1971. *J. Exptl. Med. Suppl.,* in press.

Taylor, R. B., 1969. Cellular cooperation in the antibody response of mice to two serum albumins: Specific function of thymus cells. *Transplant. Rev.* **1**:114.

Turk, J. L., and Humphrey, J. H., 1961. Immunological unresponsiveness in guinea pigs. II. The effect of unresponsiveness on the development of delayed type hypersensitivity to protein antigens. *Immunology* **4**:310.

Unanue, E. R., and Askonas, B. A., 1968. The immune response of mice to antigen in macrophages. *Immunology* **15**:287.

Unanue, E. R., and Cerottini, J. C., 1970. The function of macrophage in the immune response. *Seminars Hematol.* 7:225.

Weigle, W. O., 1961. The immune response of rabbits tolerant to bovine serum albumin to the injection of other heterologous serum albumins. *J. Exptl. Med.* 114:111.

Weigle, W. O., 1962. Termination of acquired immunological tolerance to protein antigens following immunization with altered protein antigens. *J. Exptl. Med.* 116:913.

Weigle, W. O., 1964. Studies on the termination of acquired tolerance to serum protein antigens following injection of serologically related antigens. *Immunology* 7:239.

Weigle, W. O., 1965. The induction of autoimmunity in rabbits following injection of heterologous or altered homologous thyroglobulin. *J. Exptl. Med.* 121:289.

Chapter 7

Application of Marrow Grafts in Human Disease: Its Problems and Potential

George W. Santos

Division of Oncology
Department of Medicine
The Johns Hopkins University and Oncology Service
Baltimore City Hospitals
Baltimore, Maryland

INTRODUCTION

The present chapter is not intended as an exhaustive review of marrow transplantation but is rather a somewhat personal view distilled from more than 15 years of laboratory and clinical work. In the following pages, the rationale for, problems associated with, and current results of clinical marrow transplantation for bone marrow failure, organ grafting, and malignancy will be outlined.

The initial discovery of Jacobson *et al.* (1949) that mice could be protected from an otherwise lethal dose of X-ray by the simple device of lead-shielding the spleen led to the subsequent observations of others that a variety of lethally X-irradiated mammals could be saved from death by the intravenous injection of syngeneic, allogeneic, or, in some cases, xenogeneic marrow suspensions (van Bekkum and deVries, 1967). Under these conditions, the injected marrow cells do not "home" to the appropriate organs of derivation but lodge in a variety of tissues. The vigor of their continued growth and function in a particular tissue will depend upon the local microenvironment. Once equilibrium is reached, it is found that the recipient's hematopoietic and

Supported in part by a National Cancer Institute Grant (CA-06973), and a National Institute of Allergy and Infectious Diseases Contract (PH 43-66-924).

lymphopoietic compartments are largely or completely replaced by the appropriate cell type derived from the marrow donor (van Bekkum and deVries, 1967). These initial observations provided the laboratory worker with the stimulus and much of the methodology for further fundamental investigations of the differentiation and kinetics of hematopoietic stem cells, kinetics of antibody formation, thymus-marrow interactions, etc. The clinician was no less excited by these early studies because of the obvious possibilities of application to human disease; however, the majority of early clinical attempts at marrow grafting failed because of inadequate immunosuppression, administration of too little marrow, failure to recognize that transfusions before grafting may presensitize to donor antigens, failure to adequately prevent or manage the intensity of graft *vs.* host (GVH), disease, failure to provide adequate supportive care for patients with marrow aplasia, and finally poor selection of patients, many of whom were grossly infected or moribund at the time of the procedure (Bortin, 1970). Because of these failures, the initial enthusiasm was chilled and activity in this area was sporadic over the subsequent years. Recently, however, new knowledge in the areas of HL-A tissue typing, immunosuppression, prevention of severe GVH disease and immunological deficiency diseases, and patient supportive care (newer isolation techniques, platelet and white blood cell administration, use of antibiotics and antifungal agents) has led to a renewed enthusiasm in several centers for the application of marrow grafts to a variety of human diseases (Congdon, 1970).

Some understanding of the development and complexities of the lymphohematopoietic system is necessary if we are to logically apply marrow transplants in human disease. Current information, largely derived from the mouse, indicates that the lymphohematopoietic system in the mammal originates with primordial stem cells first found in the yolk sac. Cells migrate from there to the epithelial structures of the thymus, to the liver, and to the bone marrow and spleen. After the neonatal period, most of the pluripotent stem cells (cells which are capable of differentiating toward hematopoietic or lymphoid lines) reside in the marrow.

For purposes of clarity it is useful to view the interactions of the hematopoietic and lymphopoietic systems in a somewhat oversimplified way, as illustrated in Fig. 1 (Cooper *et al.*, 1967; Good *et al.*, 1967; Möller, 1969). Pluripotential stem cells (P cells) are present in the marrow that may give rise to hematopoietic stem cells (H cells) or lymphoid stem cells (L cells). H cells leave the marrow via the blood to take residence in the spleen and occasionally the liver. These cells under the appropriate stimulus (primarily in the marrow) will differentiate into the more specialized granulocytes, erythrocytes, and megakaryocytes.

The L cells may become bone marrow-derived lymphocytes, the so-called B lymphocytes, under the still undefined bursal equivalent in mammals.

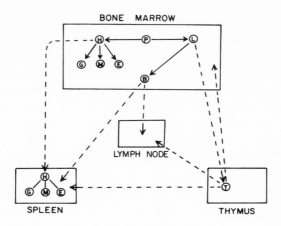

Figure 1. A highly schematic representation of the lymphohematopoietic system. P, pluripotential stem cell; H, hematopoietic stem cell; L, lymphoid stem cell; B, bone marrow–derived lymphocyte; T, thymus–derived lymphocyte; G, granulocyte; M, megakaryocyte; E, erythrocyte. Solid lines with arrows represent differentiation. Broken lines with arrows represent migration.

The B lymphocytes are highly specialized for eventual humoral antibody production requiring or not requiring the cooperation of thymus-derived lymphocytes (depending upon the antigen). Some of these B cells migrate directly to the spleen, lymph nodes, and peritoneal cavity. In the lymphatic tissues the B lymphocytes, which are short-lived compared to thymus-derived lymphocytes, occupy the outer cortex and medulla of lymph nodes as well as the periphery of spleen follicles and germinal centers.

The L cells may also migrate to the thymus or come under its humoral influence to differentiate into thymus-derived or T lymphocytes. The T lymphocytes will also migrate to the peripheral lymphatic tissues, where they occupy the paracortical regions of the lymph nodes and periarteriolar areas of the spleen follicles and comprise a highly mobile population found in high concentration in the thoracic duct lymph and peripheral blood. The T lymphocytes constitute the long-lived population and the cells of immunological memory. Apart from their role in the cooperation with B lymphocytes for certain types of humoral responses, they appear to be the cells involved with the expression of cellular immunity.

Most of the information regarding T and B lymphocytes has been derived from studies in mouse strains where bone marrow preparations contain very few T lymphocytes. Marrow from such strains of mice does not cause severe GVH disease in adult thymectomized allogeneic mice given lethal doses of X-ray, presumably because there is no thymus to generate thymus-derived cells (Van Putten, 1964). However, marrow from other strains of mice under these conditions may produce severe GVH disease, presumably because of the presence of T lymphocytes in the inocula (Simmons *et al.*, 1965). Similarly, adult thymectomized rats given allogeneic marrow following the administration of a lethal dose of cyclophosphamide (CY) will show a GVH disease as severe as that seen in sham-thymectomized controls (Uy and Santos, unpublished observations). In addition, adult thymectomized Lewis rats given syngeneic marrow after a lethal dose of CY recover their ability to make antibody to sheep erythrocytes or reject allogeneic skin grafts at the same time as sham-operated controls (Uy and Santos, unpublished observations). Furthermore, histoincompatible marrow given to lethally irradiated or CY-treated rats, dogs, primates, and man produces GVH disease of much earlier onset and intensity than is usually observed in the mouse (van Bekkum and deVries, 1967; Thomas *et al.*, 1962; Santos and Owens, 1968a; Santos *et al.*, 1970a).

If the duality of the lymphoid system in terms of T and B lymphocytes holds true for most mammals, it must therefore be assumed that in certain strains of mice and in rats, dogs, primates, and man a fair number of T lymphocytes return to establish residence in the marrow. Recent studies of specific membrane markers for T and B lymphocytes (discussed at length by Nussenzweig and Pincus in Chapter 4) should provide the techniques for directly answering this question.

The most logical application of marrow grafts would seem to be in those situations where there is failure of the P, H, or L cells to perform their function either because of "experiments of nature" or because of external factors often created by man himself. One must recognize, however, the concept of at least two possibilities whenever a clinical situation appears wherein there appears to be a functional defect related to the marrow. Is the functional defect in question due to a failure of the microenvironment or is it due to an actual defect in the cell itself? Marrow transplantation is logical in the latter situation but not in the former.

Marrow transplantation has potential application in preparing individuals for organ grafting from the same donor and application in the treatment of certain forms of malignancy. The rationale for these approaches will be discussed below.

FAILURE OF THE PLURIPOTENTIAL CELL (P CELL)

No proven examples of failure of the P cell exist in animal models or in human disease. Indeed such conditions, if they do occur, are probably incompatible with life. There is a condition, however, where infants born with a form of lymphopenic thymic dysplasia have an additional defect, aleukocytosis. This condition has been termed *reticular dysgenesia* (deVaal and Seynhaeve, 1959; Gitlin *et al.*, 1964). Because these children have died in the first days of life, it has not been possible to obtain adequate information about their hematopoietic and lymphoid systems. Morphologically, these children are extremely deficient in lymphatic and hematopoietic tissues. It has been suggested that this disorder involves a failure of the P cell to differentiate toward the H- and L-cell lines (Hoyer *et al.*, 1967). If the suggestion is true, the question remains as to whether or not we are dealing with a true cellular defect or a defect in the microenvironment. A marrow transplant in this situation might well clarify the issue.

FAILURE OF THE IMMUNE SYSTEM (L CELL)

Thymectomy in the newborn mouse has profound effects on the development of the immune system. In this situation, the absence of the appropriate microenvironment (thymus influence) precludes the development of thymus-derived lymphocytes. Neither thymus extracts nor thymus cell suspensions restore neonatally thymectomized animals to normal immunological reactivity. If such mice are grafted with intact thymus tissue, however, they have a normal life span, normally developed lymphoid tissues, and normal immune mechanisms. In such situations, most of the lymphoid cells multiplying in the spleen and thymus implant are of host (not donor) origin (Miller, 1964). This latter observation and the requirements of an intact thymus structure lend support to the notion that it is the epithelial structures of the thymus that are important for the development of the T lymphocyte.

The neonatally thymectomized mouse may represent a model for a clinical entity—congenital absence of the thymus and parathyroid glands with aortic arch anomaly, as described by DiGeorge (1967). Children with this apparently nonheritable syndrome fail to show any evidence of cellular immunity. They fail to show skin reactivity to a variety of bacterial, fungal, and viral antigens. Delayed hypersensitivity to skin sensitizers cannot be induced in them, and normal lymphocytes from skin-positive individuals cannot transfer positivity to them. Furthermore, their lymphocytes fail to respond to phytohemagglutin (PHA) in culture, and allogeneic skin grafts are not rejected.

Immunoglobulin and lymphocyte levels may be normal and plasma cells present. Whether or not such patients can synthesize antibody of some types is not altogether clear. Deliberate immunization has consistently failed to yield detectable antibody, yet these individuals may demonstrate low levels of persistent agglutinating antibody to blood groups A and B, *Escherichia coli*, and

Candida. Do these levels of antibody provide a clue to what antigens are thymus-independent in man? Are they related to antibody produced by a small population of maternal lymphocytes that have been demonstrated to persist in some patients with DiGeorge syndrome (DiGeorge, 1967)?

Although the histology of lymphoid structures may be modified by the recurrent infections that plague these patients, the available data indicate a depletion of cellularity in thymus-dependent areas with the sparing of a whole system of lymphocytes, germinal centers, and plasma cells, presumably the marrow-derived lymphocytic system.

Thymus rather than marrow transplants would seem to be quite logical in this condition, and in two instances where this has been attempted delayed hypersensitivity and lymphocyte transformability were rapidly restored (August *et al.*, 1968; Cleveland *et al.*, 1968). In both instances theoretical and practical problems were encountered. Nevertheless, these initial attempts were encouraging. The absence of donor-type lymphocytes in the blood of these patients after thymus transplantation was, of course, what was to be expected from the experimental work of Miller (1964).

It is interesting to speculate whether or not sufficient numbers of T lymphocytes might be transplanted with marrow in the human to repair, at least temporarily, the immunological defect in DiGeorge syndrome. A marrow transplant would not seem to hold any advantage over a thymus transplant except that of ease of procurement. On the other hand, the risk of GVH would seem to be greater with a marrow transplant than with a thymus implant (Owens and Santos, 1968). Although there is no apparent stem cell defect associated with the DiGeorge syndrome, one cannot be totally convinced until such patients have been demonstrated on long term follow-up to be restored to normal immunological capacity with only thymus transplants.

Although GVH has not been described in DiGeorge syndrome, it has been seen in the combined immunological deficiency syndromes (see below) following ordinary blood transfusions (Hathaway *et al.*, 1967; Hong *et al.*, 1968) or has occurred as a result of probable maternal to fetal transfusions *in utero* (Hathaway *et al.*, 1965a,b; Dooren *et al.*, 1968; Kadowaki *et al.*, 1965; Shapiro, 1967). In this regard, it is of interest that 2% female cells were seen on karyotype analysis of the first case (a male) of DiGeorge syndrome (DiGeorge, 1967). These female cells must have resulted from a maternal to fetal transfusion. Why there was no evidence of GVH disease in this child and in a case of thymic alymphoplasia in a male child with female (presumably maternal) cells (Githens *et al.*, 1969) is not known. Were there too few female cells to give rise to a recognizable GVH reaction or was there a maternal humoral mechanism for blocking the reaction of maternal cells against the child's tissues, as has recently been described by Hellström *et al.* (1969)?

There are certain combined immune deficiency syndromes in which there is no demonstrable ability to make antibody or express cellular immune reactions, with varying degrees of lymphopenia and different modes of inheritance (Hitzig and Willi, 1961; Olson *et al.*, 1967; Miller and Schieken, 1967; Bergsma and Good, 1967). It has been suggested that some of these diseases arise from a primary defect in the P cell to differentiate to the L cell or in a primary defect in the L cell itself (Hoyer *et al.*, 1967). Indeed, some therapeutic effect has been seen with marrow grafts from histocompatible siblings (Hitzig and Willi, 1961; Meuwissen *et al.*, 1969, 1971; DeKoning *et al.*, 1969). One of the reported cases was the sex-linked form of lymphopenic hypogammaglobulinemia (Meuwissen *et al.*, 1969), and two were the autosomal recessive form (Swiss type) (Meuwissen *et al.*, 1971, DeKoning *et al.*, 1969).

There are a number of other conditions that could be classified as immunological deficiency diseases that may represent failure of a differentiative pathway of the L cell by virtue of a cellular defect or of a microenvironment defect. Unfortunately, however, the description, classification, and understanding of these diseases are still far from complete (Kay, 1970). Nevertheless, marrow transplantation has been attempted in two of these disease syndromes.

The Wiskott-Aldrich syndrome (sex-linked recessive) is characterized by recurrent pyogenic injections, eczema, and thrombocytopenia (Wiskott, 1937; Aldrich *et al.*, 1954). Patients with this syndrome have lymphopenia, lack delayed hypersensitivity as assayed by skin tests, and have defective lymphocyte blastogenesis *in vitro* in response to PHA, and to specific antigens (Oppenheim *et al.*, 1970). These patients also have a defective humoral antibody response to carbohydrate but not to protein antigen (Cooper *et al.*, 1968). The lack of antibodies to carbohydrate antigens is thought to be due to a failure to process the antigen, presumably by macrophages (Cooper *et al.*, 1968).

Douglas and Fudenberg (1969) described a patient with Wiskott-Aldrich syndrome who at the age of 2 years was admitted for therapy on a regimen of monthly plasma infusions first from his father and later from his mother. A syndrome developed that was highly suggestive of GVH disease, and it was suggested that this might have been caused by the engraftment of maternal lymphocytes contaminating the plasma infusions. No direct proof for this hypothesis was available, however.

Bach *et al.* (1968) transplanted marrow from an HL-A matched sibling in this condition without preparing the recipient with immunosuppressive treatment. The graft failed to take. Subsequently, another graft was attempted with the same donor, but this time a CY dose and dose schedule as outlined by Santos *et al.* (1970*b*) were employed as immunosuppressive therapy for the recipient. The patient experienced a dramatic clinical improvement and remained well for at least 24 months thereafter. Platelet levels, however, have not increased markedly, and karyotype analysis indicates that donor lympho-cytes (female) constitute about 20% of the lymphocytes in the blood. Marrow karyotypes are all recipient (male) in type (Bach, personal communication). A number of questions are raised: (1) Why was immunosuppression required for a marrow take in this last case? The case described by Douglas and Fudenberg (1969) suggests that it was not required in their patient. (2) Why wasn't the patient of Bach *et al.* (1968) presensitized by the prior marrow infusion with subsequent failure of the second graft despite immunosuppressive treatment? (CY will not eliminate the presensitized state.) (3) By what mechanism was the patient of Bach *et al.* (1968) improved? Was the improvement due to transfer factor (Lawrence and Valentine, 1970) that has been reported at least partially to repair this condition (Levin *et al.*, 1970) or was it due to the few donor lymphocytes that enjoyed long-term engraftment?

Mucocutaneous candidiasis is a chronic infection by *Candida albicans* involving the skin, nails, scalp, and buccal and vaginal mucous membranes (Winner and Hurley, 1964). Many patients with this disease fail to exhibit cutaneous cellular hypersensitivity to the causative organism, although they are capable of specific immunoglobulin production (Chilgren *et al.*, 1967; Imperato *et al.*, 1968). Lymphocytes from these patients are usually capable of blast transformation in response to PHA and in some cases to *Candida* antigen (Chilgren *et al.*, 1969; Marmor and Barnett, 1968), even though these patients do not exhibit delayed hypersensitivity skin reactions.

Buckley *et al.* (1968) reported immunological reconstitution of a patient with chronic mucocutaneous candidiasis and staphylococcal botryomycosis by means of a bone marrow transplant without preceding immunosuppressive therapy. Delayed hypersensitivity to *Candida* and two other antigens was de-tected 6 months after transplant, and good therapeutic results were said to have resulted for both infections. There was no evidence in this patient, how-ever, for persistence of the infused marrow cells.

Rocklin *et al.* (1970) noted that lymphocytes from two anergic patients with chronic mucocutaneous candidiasis failed to produce macrophage migra-tion inhibition factor (MIF), a mediator associated with delayed hypersensi-tivity, following antigenic challenge. After the administration of transfer factor dialysate, one patient was able to manifest cutaneous hypersensitivity to *Candida*, and her lymphocytes were able to respond to this antigen by MIF production. In light of these results, one may wonder if the patient described by Buckley *et al.* (1968) was benefited primarily by transfer factor carried along with the marrow allograft. This cannot be the entire explanation, how-ever, since the authors were able to induce delayed hypersensitivity to a contact allergen after the transplant. Transfer factor can only transfer the reactivity of the donor and not the ability to be sensitized (Lawrence and Valentine, 1970).

Further questions are raised about the syndrome of mucocutaneous candidiasis in the report of Canales *et al.* (1969). These authors studied an anergic patient with this syndrome whose cells responded *in vitro* to stimulation with PHA but not with mumps or monilia antigen. Cells of the patient neither responded nor stimulated in a one-way mixed lymphocyte culture (MLC). The patient's serum inhibited the proliferative response of normal control lymphocytes stimulated with *Candida* and mumps antigen and allogeneic cells. These abnormal results appeared to be the result of the serum factor inhibiting the blastogenic response of the T lymphocyte. The defect appeared to be genetic in this patient, as there were other affected members of the family. This case appears to be different than the two described above. One wonders whether or not transfer factor would have caused a repair of cellular reactivity in this patient and whether or not the serum factor in this patient would have inhibited MIF production in normal lymphocytes.

It is clear that there are a variety of conditions wherein there are functional defects in the lymphoid system. In some of these situations, enough is known to rationally approach therapy with or without marrow transplants as is indicated. In the bulk of these conditions, however, not enough is known. The continued unraveling of these various disease states remains one of the most challenging and exciting areas of cellular biology.

FAILURE OF THE HEMATOPOIETIC SYSTEM (H CELL)

Failure of the hematopoietic microenvironment may result from the lack of important local stromal factors as well as a more general deficiency in terms of hormones (as in Addison's disease, Simmond's disease, or hypothyroidism [Wintrobe, 1967]), natural poietins (such as erythropoietin, in the anephric state [Wintrobe, 1967]), or nutritional requirements (iron, vitamin B_{12}, etc.). In the broadest sense, failure of the microenvironment would also include situations where noxious factors are operative, such as infectious agents (as in miliary tuberculosis [Wintrobe, 1967], equine infectious anemia [Peters, 1945], hepatitis [Levy *et al.*, 1965], etc.), chemical agents (gold, benzol, etc.), physical agents (radium, strontium-90, etc.), or immunological factors operative in certain autoimmune conditions. Many of the causes of microenvironment failure have been known for some time, and are trivial and easily correctable (i.e., deficiency diseases), while the causes of others have been more occult but nevertheless have been explained after intensive and often brilliant investigation. An example of the latter is well illustrated by those cases of erythrocytic aplasia described by Krantz and Kao (1967). These workers were able to demonstrate the presence of a 7S-immunoglobulin in the serum of patients afflicted with this disease that specifically inhibited the proliferation and maturation of cells of the erythrocytic series. Further, they showed that this autoimmune state was reversible when patients were given tolerable doses of immunosuppressive drugs.

The concept of the stromal microenvironment determining hematopoietic differentiation has gained considerable support from studies of mice with mutations at the W and Sl loci (Russell, 1963). Mice of genotype Sl/Sl^d or W/W^v are markedly anemic, have no pigment-producing cells in their skin, and are sterile. The bases for these defects are different for each of the mutations. The W/W^v mice have defective hematopoietic stem cells (McCulloch et al., 1964) as well as defective pigment-producing cells (Mayer and Green, 1968). In Sl/Sl^d mice there is a defect in the microenvironment which prevents hematopoiesis (McCulloch et al., 1965) and pigment production. In both conditions, the L cell and its microenvironment appear to be intact (Mekori and Phillips, 1969).

The Sl/Sl^d mouse, as mentioned previously, provides a relatively clear example of a situation in which the microenvironment for hematopoiesis is genetically defective while the H cell itself appears normal. Recently, it has been reported that such mice may be restored to normal by grafts of spleen stroma which are able to provide the proper microenvironment for hematopoiesis (Bernstein, 1970). This latter observation is of great interest and offers therapeutic possibilities for the as yet to be discovered human counterpart of the Sl/Sl^d model.

The W/W^v mouse provides perhaps the best model of marrow failure due to an H-cell defect (Russell, 1963; McCulloch et al., 1964). Indeed, the defective hematopoiesis in these mice has been repaired by allogeneic marrow transplants following whole-body X-irradiation (Russell et al., 1956).

Ionizing radiation as well as a variety of cytotoxic agents are capable of producing lethal effects by destroying or at least severely injuring the H cell. The transplantation of syngeneic marrow has effectively reversed these lethal effects in many instances (van Bekkum and deVries, 1967). In some situations, allogeneic marrow has also been able to reverse these effects following X-ray (van Bekkum and deVries, 1967) and the alkylating agents aminochlorambucil (Beilby et al., 1960; Stewart, 1964), and CY (Santos et al., 1970b; Santos, 1967a; Santos and Owens, 1969). Although marrow infusions have successfully reversed potentially lethal doses of ionizing radiation in reactor accidents (Jammet et al., 1959; Thomas et al., 1971a) or in therapeutic misadventure with cytotoxic agents (Beilby et al., 1960), the greatest incidence of potentially fatal aplasia with X-ray and cytotoxic agents is seen under conditions where the aplasia is induced intentionally for the purposes of marrow grafting; accordingly, this aspect of the subject will be discussed later at some length.

In the preceding discussion of the microenvironment, it was noted that a variety of chemical and physical agents may be causally related to aplasia.

However, about 50% of all cases of aplasia have no known cause (Scott *et al.*, 1959). *A priori*, in most of these situations one does not know with any degree of certainty whether the persisting defect is in the microenvironment or in the H cell itself. Some insight into this question has been provided, however, by clinical studies wherein various forms of aplasia have been corrected by marrow infusions.

At least ten patients with aplasia have received syngeneic (i.e., identical twin) marrow transplants. Three died before the effect of the infusion could be evaluated, and two were not benefited by the procedure. Five patients recovered completely, and the time of recovery after infusion indicated successful marrow transplantation. Of the successful cases, three were due to unknown causes, one followed chloramphenicol, and one followed the administration of anticonvulsant drugs (Pillow *et al.*, 1966).

Amiel *et al.* (1970) reported successful partial but persistent allogeneic marrow takes that dramatically improved the clinical status of the patients in one case of idiopathic aplasia, in one case following chloramphenicol, and in one case following hepatitis. No evidence of a take was demonstrated in four other cases of idiopathic aplasia. Immunosuppression was provided by pretreatment with an antilymphocyte globulin (ALG) fraction. Rogentine *et al.* (1970), using the same ALG preparation, also reported a partial take of allogeneic marrow in a case of idiopathic aplasia. Meuwissen *et al.* (1971) were unable to demonstrate an allogeneic marrow take in two patients with idiopathic aplasia. Transplantation was attempted twice in one patient, the first time employing antilymphocyte serum, prednisone, and azathioprine as immunosuppression and the second time employing CY. The second patient was given CY for immunosuppression. It should be noted that in both of these cases the bulk of the marrow was administered intraperitoneally, a route shown to be inferior to the intravenous route (van Bekkum and deVries, 1967). Furthermore, these patients died at 3 days and 10 days after grafting, a time that may be too early to adequately assess the presence or absence of a marrow take.

The results reported above are encouraging and clearly demonstrate that in some cases of idiopathic aplasia, in some following chloramphenicol, and in some following hepatitis the causative agent is no longer operative and the resulting defect resides in the H cell rather than in the microenvironment. The reported failures do not rule out the possibility that a stem cell defect was operative in some of the cases, since immunosuppression may not have been adequate in these patients, many of whom may have been presensitized to major or minor transplantation antigens of their donor because of preceding blood transfusions.

Fanconi's syndrome (Wintrobe, 1967) or congenital pancytopenia is a condition wherein there are varying degrees of pancytopenia. Other features of the disorder include dwarfism, microcephaly, and hypogenitalism. The etiology of the disorder is unknown, but it is generally believed to be hereditary, perhaps due to a recessive gene, or the result of reciprocal chromosomal translocation in one of the parents and a duplication deficiency in the affected offspring. Cytogenetic studies have revealed a variety of structural aberrations and a specific type of polyploidy. Although it is possible that this disease is due to an H-cell defect, it is also possible that it may represent a failure of the complete hematopoietic microenvironment. Marrow transplantation in this disease would undoubtedly yield interesting clues as to its true etiology.

Apart from disorders of the H cell itself, there may be cellular defects in the erythrocyte, granulocyte, or megakaryocyte cell lines. In many instances, cellular defects are suspected in the clinical hemoglobinopathies, congenital spherocytosis, or the flextail mutation in mice, where the mutation affects differentiation of erythropoietic cells but has no effect on the production of granulocytes (Thompson et al., 1966). In a number of instances, however, the available evidence does not allow one to discriminate between cellular defects independent of the microenvironment or defects of the microenvironment that may be private to a given line of differentiated hematopoietic cells. A condition has been described, for instance, of an anemic individual whose plasma contained no transferrin (Heilmeyer, 1966). This person might have been classed as having a type of idiopathic anemia possibly related to a cellular defect in the erythrocyte series had levels of transferrin not been determined. It is interesting to speculate that a marrow graft nevertheless may have repaired the anemia, since cells derived from marrow infusions are capable of producing transferrin (Phillips and Thorbecke, 1966).

In principle, it would seem logical to attempt marrow transplantation in the more severe forms of the hemoglobinopathies such as sickle cell anemia and certain types of the thalassemias. Except for a few unsuccessful attempts recently (Congdon, 1970), transplantation for these disorders has not been pursued in the past. Although these diseases may be severe, the prognosis is much better than that of aplastic anemia, acute leukemia, and some of the immunological deficiency diseases. Success with marrow transplantation in these latter areas undoubtedly will see an increase in the therapeutic trials in sickle cell anemia and thalassemia.

MARROW TRANSPLANTATION AS A PRELUDE TO ORGAN GRAFTING

The successful transplantation of allogeneic or even xenogeneic marrow allows the permanent survival of other tissue grafts from the same donor

(Mathé *et al.*, 1963) or, in the case of inbred animals, from the same inbred strain (van Bekkum and deVries, 1967). Rats (Santos, 1967a) and mice (Santos and Owens, 1969) given allogeneic marrow or lymphohematopoietic cells following CY will accept both host- and donor-type skin while rejecting third-party skin. Lewis inbred rats pretreated with CY followed by marrow grafts from $LBNF_1$ rats become stable chimeras and will accept $LBNF_1$ kidneys (Guttman *et al.*, unpublished observations). Indeed, even mice given rat bone marrow following lethal irradiation will accept subcutaneously placed grafts of rat pulmonary tissue (Santos *et al.*, 1960). At the present time, however, this offers only a hope for the future use in the clinic because of the as yet unresolved hazards associated with marrow grafting in man.

What has been stated above generally appears to hold true; however, it has been pointed out by Boyse *et al.* (1971) and Lance *et al.* (1971) that chimerism in man, cattle, mice, and rats does not always guarantee the survival of skin allografts from the donor whose hematopoietic cells continue to colonize the recipient. These authors were able to show that C57BL/6 mice or DBA/2 mice made "complete" lymphohematopoietic chimeras by the infusion of $(C57BL/6 \times A)F_1$ or $(BALB/c \times DBA/2)F_1$ marrow or spleen cells, respectively, following lethal irradiation were able to reject A or BALB/c strain skin grafts. On the basis of these studies, these workers have suggested that epidermal cells contain distinctive transplantation alloantigens not also possessed by marrow and lymphoid cells. They inferred that the maintenance of tolerance of self-skin alloantigen was lost when the immunocompetent cell population was removed from the environment where this antigen is normally present. Unfortunately, these authors did not graft these animals with host-type skin to rule out the possibility of a nonspecific effect of the chimeric state.

The idea of tissue-specific alloantigens may or may not turn out to be trivial in man, and therefore it is hoped that further experimentation will further define this concept both in theoretical as well as in practical terms.

MARROW TRANSPLANTATION IN THE TREATMENT OF MALIGNANCY

In theory, there are at least three reasons why one might wish to employ marrow transplantation in malignancy: (1) to provide the means of administering doses of anticancer agents in what would ordinarily be lethal doses were it not for the protection afforded by transplanted marrow, (2) to provide specific immunotherapy by the transplantation of syngeneic marrow, and (3) to provide a therapeutic effect by means of a mild or controlled GVH reaction utilizing allogeneic marrow.

For purposes of discussion, it is useful to consider that tumor cells may offer normal as well as tumor-specific transplantation antigens as potential targets for reactive lymphoid cells or cytotoxic antibody. Lymphoid-derived and leukemic tumor cells are relatively rich in normal transplantation antigens, while nonlymphoid-derived tumors such as fibrosarcoma and adenocarcinoma tumors may be relatively poor in such antigens. On the other hand, the strength of tumor-specific transplantation antigens will vary from tumor to tumor.

USE OF SYNGENEIC MARROW WHERE TUMOR-SPECIFIC ANTIGENS ARE WEAK OR IN DOUBT

The first attempt to treat a malignancy by irradiation and marrow transplantation was made by Hollcroft *et al.* (1953), who used a transplantable leukemia in inbred guinea pigs. Animals carrying the leukemia were exposed to irradiation followed by the infusion of syngeneic marrow. Remissions were noted, but no permanent cures were obtained. The duration of remission appeared within experimental limits to be linearly related to the dose of radiation employed. These disappointing results were subsequently confirmed by many other workers (van Bekkum and deVries, 1967) and stand in contrast to the initially exciting report by Barnes *et al.* (1956). These authors reported a considerable number of cures in mice carrying a transplantable lymphosarcoma following irradiation with a dose of 1500 r given over 25 hr, followed by the infusion of syngeneic marrow. These workers were unable to repeat these observations (Barnes and Loutit, 1957). In general, most workers have failed to find much of a therapeutic effect using this approach.

A similar failure to show a marked effect of this approach in the clinic has been noted by Thomas *et al.* (1971*a*), who reported three patients with acute leukemia who were given 800-1000 rad whole-body irradiation followed by marrow from an identical twin. These patients recovered from the irradiation, but leukemia recurred 48-84 days later. A fourth patient was given 1596 rad and syngeneic marrow and showed hematopoietic recovery but died early after the transplant of hepatic failure, presumably due to viral hepatitis.

USE OF SYNGENEIC MARROW WHERE STRONG TUMOR ANTIGENS EXIST OR ARE SUSPECTED

Trentin (1957) reported some success employing the transplantable Gardner lymphosarcoma in mice. Ten of eleven C3H mice, irradiated and treated with syngeneic marrow on the day of inoculation of the tumor, were alive after 190 days. deVries and Vos (1958, 1960) have also reported a significant prolongation of life and even long-term survival of C57BL and (CBA × C57BL)F$_1$ mice carrying a transplantable lymphosarcoma, following lethal irradiation and transplantation of syngeneic marrow and syngeneic lymphoid cells. As discussed by van Bekkum and deVries (1967), the beneficial effect of the treatments given by Trentin (1957) and deVries and Vos (1958, 1960) were probably due to the antigenicity of the tumor cells. This seems quite likely, since it has been shown that the dose of X-ray required to sterilize an *in vitro* suspension of murine leukemic cells extends into the range of X-ray dose that will produce irreversible CNS damage (van Bekkum and deVries, 1967).

Even with tumors that possess known and strong tumor-specific antigens there usually has been a failure to demonstrate a marked therapeutic effect with whole-body X-ray (Floersheim, 1969) or CY (Owens, 1970; Fefer, 1970) followed by the administration of syngeneic lymphohematopoietic cells.

Floersheim (1969) treated mice bearing well-established Moloney lymphoma tumor with single high doses of dimethyl myleran, whose otherwise lethal effects were abrogated by the injection of syngeneic marrow. More than one half of the animals so treated enjoyed tumor-free remissions lasting more than 150 days. Dimethyl myleran has not been immunosuppressive in his studies (Floersheim and Ruszkiewcz, 1969), and tumor-specific antigens have been demonstrated for the Moloney lymphoma (Klein *et al.*, 1966). The success of this form of therapy therefore depended upon a synergism between the antitumor action of the drug and the immunological resistance of the host to tumor-specific antigens. In this context, it is to be noted that lethal irradiation and marrow transplantation did not give results anywhere as comparable, presumably because of the immunosuppressive action of X-ray. It would seem, therefore, that if one is dealing with a highly antigenic tumor, syngeneic marrow transplantation might show a reasonable therapeutic effect, if the antitumor agent employed for lowering the tumor burden is not immunosuppressive (i.e., busulfan [Santos, 1966*a*], dimethyl myleran [Floersheim and Ruszkiewcz, 1969], or possibly mithramycin [Santos, 1967*b*]); alternatively, if X-ray or CY is used, supplementation of a syngeneic marrow graft with large amounts of lymphocytes from the donor might be effective.

Another approach to this problem has been to employ syngeneic lymphohematopoietic cells sensitized to putative tumor antigens. This form of immunotherapy has been reported to be successful even against established clinically detectable primary tumors induced by Moloney sarcoma virus (Fefer, 1970). In addition, Fefer (1970) was able to show an additive effect of CY treatment combined with specifically sensitized syngeneic cells in eradicating a transplantable sarcoma. The transfer of syngeneic nonimmunized spleen cells after CY treatment has no greater an effect on the outcome than that with CY alone.

Identical twin human donors have not been immunized with putative tumor antigens of their twin with malignancy for ethical reasons. Thomas *et al.* (1971*a*), however, have approached this problem in a unique way. Tumor cells of three patients with acute leukemia and one with lymphosarcoma were collected and stored in dimethyl sulfoxide (DMSO) at -180 C prior to treatment. These patients received 1000 rad of whole-body irradiation followed by the infusion of 12 to 25 × 10^9 nucleated bone marrow cells from an identical twin. Each patient also received 4 units of buffy coat cells containing lymphocytes and platelets three times weekly for 3 weeks. In addition, each patient was given subcutaneous once weekly injections of autologous tumor cells irradiated with 10,000 rad *in vitro*. A patient with lymphoblastic leukemia had a recurrence of disease and died 33 days later; another patient with leukemia showed recovery but died 6 weeks later of a progressive interstitial pneumonia of unknown cause. At autopsy there was no evidence of leukemia. The third patient, with acute myelogenous leukemia, was in complete remission for 8 months and then developed progressive marrow aplasia with the definite reappearance of leukemia after 11 months. The fourth patient, with lymphosarcoma, showed hematopoietic recovery and is without evidence of disease 105 days following transplantation. The true effectiveness of this interesting therapeutic approach can only be judged after further clinical trial.

USE OF ALLOGENEIC MARROW WITH HISTOINCOMPATIBLE DONORS

Studies in a variety of animals and in man have shown that the major transplantation antigens are controlled by genes at one chromosomal locus designated *H-2* for the mouse, *AgB* for the rat, *DL-A* for the dog, and *HL-A* for man. In inbred mice, for instance, allogeneic pairs of animals may share the same *H-2* alleles but differ genetically by virtue of loci controlling the expression of minor transplant antigens. For purposes of discussion, such animals will be called *histocompatible* as opposed to *syngeneic* wherein all major and minor loci are shared. Animals differing at the major *H-2* loci will be called *histoincompatible*. In outbred species such as the dog and man, genetic analysis of the typing data in a family permits the recognition of allogeneic siblings who differ by two alleles or one allele or who are identical for both parental alleles (Bach, 1970). The latter will be called *histocompatible* and the two former *histoincompatible*.

Lethal doses of whole-body X-irradiation (van Bekkum and deVries, 1967) or high but nonlethal doses of CY (Owens, 1970) followed by allogeneic bone marrow and lymphoid cells have been employed to treat rodent lymphoid tumors and leukemias. In most studies there was a marked antitumor effect, and a few animals were able to survive free of tumor (van Bekkum and deVries, 1967); however, the majority died of GVH disease. Effective treatment of the GVH disease increased the number of tumor-free survivors (Owens, 1970; Boranić, 1968). In one study, GVH disease was controlled by CY administered after grafting, and surviving animals free of tumor were shown to be chimeras (Owens, 1970). Subsequent experiments revealed that these animals possessed both host- and donor-type lymphohematopoietic cells and thus were mixed chimeras (Owens, personal communications).

In dogs with malignant tumors, 29 histoincompatible marrow grafts were attempted following 1200 r of whole-body X-irradiation (Epstein *et al.*, 1971). Methotrexate (MTX) was administered on days, 1, 3, 6, and 11 following transplantation in an attempt to control GVH disease (Storb *et al.*, 1970*a*). Seven dogs with lymphosarcoma and one dog with anaplastic carcinoma survived beyond the first week after irradiation and demonstrated evidence of allogeneic marrow engraftment. All animals died—two following graft rejection, two with intercurrent sepsis, and three of GVH disease. The two longest survivors, dying of GVH disease on days 46 and 60, were free of clinical or histological evidence of tumor (Epstein *et al.*, 1971).

In at least two reports it was noted that severe GVH disease in mice did not produce a therapeutic effect on a fibrosarcoma and adenocarcinoma (Fefer, 1970; Santos, 1970). It has been suggested that the difference in results with lymphomas and leukemias on the one hand and these nonlymphomatous solid tumors on the other is a reflection of the relative richness of normal transplantation antigens on the surface of lymphoid-derived cells as opposed to other cells (Santos, 1970), and hence the greater susceptibility of lymphoid-derived cells to damage by GVH disease. However, in the case of a viral-induced fibrosarcoma, an antitumor effect was seen when the allogeneic donor was preimmunized with the tumor in question (Fefer, 1970). When similar experiments were performed with a spontaneously arising but transplantable fibrosarcoma and adenocarcinoma, there was no therapeutic effect on the tumor (Santos, unpublished observations). Presumably, in the first case a strong tumor-specific antigen exists but is weak or absent in the second example cited.

In general, transplantation of histoincompatible marrow following lethal whole-body irradiation in patients with leukemia has either failed to show takes or has resulted in death from GVH disease. In 21 attempts at grafting in acute leukemia, Mathé (1968) noted failure of the graft in six patients. Grafts were established in 15, eight of whom died of severe GVH disease without evidence of leukemia. Two died with a milder form of GVH disease without evidence of leukemia, and one died of varicella encephalitis 20 months after grafting, free of leukemia. This last patient had suffered from a chronic form of GVH disease, which undoubtedly increased his susceptibility to fatal infection with this virus. Four patients had very mild GVH disease and questionable persistence of donor cells. They died of recurrent leukemia.

Buckner *et al.* (1970) reported a case of a 46-year-old man with blastic crises of chronic myelogenous leukemia who was given 950 rad whole-body irradiation followed by the infusion of marrow from his sister, who differed from him by one allele controlling the expression of HL-A antigens. MTX and corticosteroids were given after grafting. GVH disease was evident by the end of the second week but appeared to be controlled. The patient died 56 days after transplant of probable cytomegalovirus infection with a complete marrow graft and no evidence of leukemia.

Amiel *et al.* (1970) attempted allogeneic histoincompatible marrow grafts in ten patients with acute leukemia who were aplastic from prior chemotherapy. These authors pretreated the recipients with horse anti-human lymphocyte globulin. Partial grafts were established in five of these cases. All five patients remained partial chimeras until recurrence of their leukemia. It is of interest that these authors stated that no GVH disease was seen in these patients. This observation and the incompleteness of chimerism was thought by these same authors to explain the recurrence of leukemia.

Santos *et al.* (1971*a*) reported the use of histoincompatible allogeneic marrow in one patient with advanced Hodgkin's disease and in two patients with acute leukemia employing CY pretreatment. All three patients showed early and severe GVH disease with onset on days 4, 5, and 6 after grafting. Patients survived for 7, 7, and 10 days after transplant. One patient died of pseudomonas infection, one died of a subarachnoid hemorrhage secondary to thrombocytopenia, and one patient died of a hemorrhagic myocarditis probably related to CY (270 mg/kg over a 10-day period). Regenerating marrow was evident in each patient, and karyotype analysis revealed marrow engraftment in one. There was no evidence of leukemia in two patients, but there were residual lesions of Hodgkin's disease in one.

USE OF ALLOGENEIC MARROW WITH HISTOCOMPATIBLE GRAFTS

Histocompatible lymphohematopoietic cells were capable of exerting a therapeutic effect on Moloney sarcoma virus-induced murine fibrosarcoma only when given after CY treatment and only if the donor had been previously immunized to the tumor antigens (Fefer, 1970). In another study, the use of nonsensitized (Santos, 1970) or sensitized (Santos, unpublished observations) histocompatible lymphohematopoietic cells was without effect when given following CY to mice bearing a transplantable (but spontaneously arising) adenocarcinoma or fibrosarcoma. There has been a paucity of other animal experiments employing histocompatible marrow, and most of the reported work has been clinical.

Thomas *et al.* (1971*b*) attempted histocompatible allogeneic marrow grafts in three individuals with acute lymphocytic leukemia, in two with acute myelogenous leukemia, in one with a blastic crisis of chronic myelogenous leukemia, and in one with Hodgkin's disease employing total body X-irradiation (1000 rad) and post-transplant treatment with MTX. There was documentation of a marrow take in three, good presumptive evidence of a take in one, and no solid evidence of a take or graft function in three. Extenuating circumstances were present in the three patients who failed to show evidence of engraftment. One patient developed severe uric acid nephropathy early after grafting as well as sepsis, and another may have been presensitized to his donor because of prior transfusions from that donor. The third failure was in a patient with the blastic crisis phase of chronic myelogenous leukemia. This patient had a very enlarged spleen, and following the marrow infusion he was found to rapidly destroy infused platelets from the marrow donor (presumably in the spleen). Perhaps the infused marrow was destroyed in the same way. One patient with Hodgkin's disease died 37 days after grafting with severe GVH disease but without evidence of residual tumor at autopsy. One patient with acute lymphocytic leukemia was noted to have transient liver abnormalities beginning 37 days after grafting (GVH disease?) which subsequently cleared. This patient has a full graft and appears to be free of his leukemia more than 400 days after transplantation (Thomas, personal communication). Two patients showed a recurrence of leukemia. One male patient with acute lymphocytic leukemia showed evidence of recurrent leukemia 24 days after transplantation. He was subsequently treated with CY (50 mg/kg for 4 consecutive days) prior to grafting with the same donor but died 14 days later with hypoplastic marrow but no evidence of leukemia. Another 15-year-old girl with acute lymphocytic leukemia received marrow from a brother. A prompt full graft was established, but leukemia recurred 62 days after transplantation. Repeated karyotype analysis, however, revealed the leukemia cells to be male (Fialkow *et al.*, 1971). This case would appear to provide strong indirect evidence for an oncogenic virus inducing a transformation in the donor's lymphocytes.

Graw *et al.* (1971) gave histocompatible allogeneic marrow to two individuals with acute lymphocytic leukemia following whole-body X-irradiation. There was no evidence for marrow engraftment in one patient who was major blood group O and who received marrow from a histocompatible sibling of major blood group A. There was evidence for marrow engraftment in the other case, but severe GVH disease began 15 days after transplant and the patient died 33 days after grafting without evidence of leukemia. It should be noted that the latter patient received multiple transfusions of platelets after grafting. These preparations were not exposed to X-irradiation, which may explain the severe early GVH disease seen in this histocompatible transplant, since platelet preparations are contaminated with lymphocytes.

Santos *et al.* (1971*a*) reported a series of histocompatible allogeneic marrow transplants in four patients with acute myelocytic leukemia and in one with acute monocytic leukemia. In two patients complete genetic analysis of the typing data was not able to confirm histocompatibility, but in each instance one allele was identified and the patient and donor were typed identically with at least 80 different anti-HL-A sera. Patients were prepared with four daily doses of CY (50-60 mg/kg per dose), and all but one patient received additional CY after grafting. Only one patient did not show evidence of engraftment but did enjoy a 3 months' remission before leukemia recurred. Moderate to severe GVH disease with onset of 20 and 30 days was seen in two patients. Relatively mild GVH disease confined to the skin was seen in one, and one patient showed no GVH disease. Two patients with grafts died at 32 and 47 days after transplant of bacterial infection. One patient died 75 days after grafting of a viral infection following severe GVH disease. This was the only patient who did not receive CY after the transplant. The course of one patient was complicated by the appearance of a diffuse interstitial pneumonitis occurring 90 days after transplantation. This condition improved on prednisone therapy, but the patient died 215 days after transplant of acute staphylococcal pneumonia. No recurrent leukemia was seen except in the patient who failed to accept his graft. Initial karyotype analysis of blood and marrow in all cases with engraftment revealed both host and donor cells. With the passage of time, however, analysis revealed only donor cells. Presumably, host lymphohematopoietic cells, perhaps damaged by CY, were "rejected" by donor cells. Table I illustrates this point in four cases.

Graw *et al.* (1971) studied seven patients with acute lymphocytic leukemia who were given 45 mg/kg of CY for 4 consecutive days prior to infusing histocompatible allogeneic marrow; MTX was administered after marrow transplantation in all but two patients. There was evidence of marrow engraftment in six patients, but, in contrast to the studies of Santos *et al.* (1971*a*), the graft was never complete in that host lymphohematopoietic cells were always present (Graw, personal communication). The one patient who failed to accept the donor's marrow was major blood group O and the donor was A. Severe GVH disease with onset 31 days after transplant was seen in one patient who died 66 days after grafting. This patient did not receive MTX after transplant and also showed no evidence of leukemia at autopsy. However, another patient also did not receive MTX after transplant and showed only mild GVH disease with onset 14 days after transplant. This patient and the remaining others (all with mild GVH disease) showed recurrent leukemia from 10 to 61 days after grafting. Where testable by karyotype analysis, the

Table I. Proof of Marrow Engraftment

Patient	Percent donor erythrocytes[a]	Number donor karyotypes/host karyotypes	
		Blood[a]	Marrow[a]
P.W.[b]	50(21), 85(25), 90(37), 100(57), 100(75)		6/3(21), 13/1(35), 20/0(75)
J.T.	30(12), 50(16), 75(30), 100(35), 100(40), 100(49)	13/1(30)	18/0(12), 12/2(21), 7/0(42)
W.E.	20(11), 25(18), 50(25)	24/3(32)	3/0(18), 15/0(32)
T.W.	20(26), 50(72), 75(92), 100(135), 100(215)	18/0(33), 20/0(47), 26/0(97), 19/0(121), 20/0(215)	21/36(16), 37/0(33), 23/0(64), 26/0(75), 3/0(121), 3/0(176), 20/0(215)

[a]Number in parentheses represents the day after transplant.
[b]Presence of donor immunoglobulin allotype by GM typing.

leukemia was shown to be of the host karyotype (Graw, personal communication). The recurrence of leukemia in these patients may possibly be related to the failure of these workers to obtain complete chimerism. It is most likely that the doses of CY were too low in these cases, as contrasted to the higher doses employed by Santos *et al.* (1971*a*). Experiments in a rodent model discussed below add credence to this suggestion.

Amato *et al.* (1971) transplanted histocompatible allogeneic marrow to two patients following CY using the drug schedule suggested by Santos *et al.* (1971*a*). The marrow was first fractionated by velocity sedimentation (Miller and Phillips, 1969) in an attempt to lessen the chances of GVH disease. The first patient, a female with acute myelogenous leukemia, died 17 days after the transplant of a ruptured mycotic aneurysm. There was no evidence of engraftment, and leukemia was noted at autopsy. The second patient, with acute lymphocytic leukemia, was treated in the same way. Marrow engraftment was demonstrated, and the patient was free of leukemia 49 days after transplant. Mild GVH disease was probably present, as evidenced by a mild skin rash occurring 23 days after transplant and an eosinophilia occurring 17 days after grafting. The efficacy of fractionated marrow in preventing GVH disease has not been demonstrated in man. Failure of engraftment in the first case may or may not be related to the way the marrow was handled during fractionation.

Meuwissen *et al.* (1971) transplanted histocompatible allogeneic marrow to a patient with advanced Hodgkin's disease following two injections of CY (50 mg/kg X 2). There was no direct evidence for engraftment, but the patient developed typical signs and symptoms (confirmed at autopsy) of GVH disease beginning 10 days after transplant. Death from bacterial sepsis occurred 27 days after the transplant. Unfortunately, no comment was made regarding the status of the Hodgkin's disease at autopsy.

Further trials of marrow transplantation in malignancy would seem warranted. The possibilities of immunizing syngeneic cells to putative tumor antigens *in vitro* or *in vivo* after the transplant are intriguing. The search for antileukemia drugs without immunosuppressive properties would also seem important in light of the work by Floersheim (1969) reported above. The results with allogeneic marrow transplantation are encouraging in terms of the antitumor effect seen in many instances. Nevertheless, the problems of GVH disease and supportive care during aplasia remain real. Finally, the possibility of a viral etiology of acute lymphocytic leukemia as suggested by the case described above from Seattle (Fialkow *et al.*, 1971) can be interpreted optimistically by those interested in bone marrow transplantation, particularly if chemical compounds are found that will block transformation by oncogenic viruses (Brockman *et al.*, 1971). Such a compound could be administered immediately following marrow transplantation.

PREPARATION OF RECIPIENTS FOR MARROW GRAFTING

In special cases of bone marrow failure where identical twins are available as donors and in situations where no immune barrier to allogeneic marrow transplantation exists, as in the autosomal recessive type of lymphopenic hypogammaglobulinemia (DeKoning *et al.*, 1969) or in the sex-linked form of this disease (Meuwissen *et al.*, 1969), no special immunosuppressive treatment of the recipient may be required; however, in these diseases it may prove to be desirable to provide the recipient with myeloablative therapy to provide "room" for the marrow graft.

If the aim is to obtain complete replacement of the lymphohematopoietic system, as might be desired in acute myelogenous leukemia, for instance, or at least partial but persistent chimerism, as may be required in the treatment of bone marrow failure or preparing for organ grafting, then one might wish to employ agents that are profoundly immunosuppressive as well as at least partially myelosuppressive. The ideal agent should be easy to administer, and of relatively short action, and one in which dose or dosimetry can be accurately calculated. Toxicity should be confined to the lymphohematopoietic system, or at least in doses used the undesired toxicity should be something that is not life-threatening and is easily managed. An additional requirement when treating malignant disease is that the agent be quite active in destroying the malignant cell. Both X-ray and CY approach but do not fully satisfy this ideal.

Ionizing radiation employed primarily in the form of whole-body X-irradiation has marked hematopoietic and immunosuppressive effects and has been until recently the only agent employed for marrow grafting. The use of whole-body X-irradiation has allowed allogeneic marrow transplantation in a variety of species and has provided us with most of what is understood about marrow transplantation today (van Bekkum and deVries, 1967).

Although X-irradiation has been used effectively to prepare recipients for marrow transplantation, its use is complicated by the production of serious injury to the entire body, which is dose-dependent. For pedagogic purposes, one can categorically divide whole-body X-irradiation injury into three types called the *hematopoietic, gastrointestinal,* and *cerebral syndromes* (van Bekkum and deVries, 1967; Smith and Congdon, 1968). These syndromes are most easily appreciated in the murine species. Mice exposed to lethal doses of X-ray up to about 1200 r regularly die between 8 to 14 days later with systemic infection as a consequence of hematopoietic failure. In the dose region of 1200–12,000 r, death is caused by irreversible damage to the gastrointestinal tract. The animals develop anorexia and excessive watery diarrhea and die between the fourth and fifth day from protein loss and fluid and electrolyte imbalance. Following doses greater than 12,000 r, the animals develop symptoms characteristic of damage to the central nervous system and death occurs within hours or at the most 1 or 2 days. The survival time has been found to decrease with increasing dose. In the mouse, a supralethal dose of X-ray may be given that will produce death of 100% of the animals, primarily from the hematopoietic syndrome. These three syndromes have been seen in other mammals such as the rat, rabbit, dog, and man, but in these animals some difficulty was encountered initially in producing just a hemato-poietic death with supralethal doses of X-ray because of overlapping of the hematopoietic and gastrointestinal syndromes. However, careful attention to dose, dose rate, and fractionation of X-ray has shown that for practical pur-poses supralethal doses of X-ray may be given to these other animals to produce primarily hematopoietic deaths. Of practical importance, however, is that the range of X-ray dose in the supralethal region that results in hemato-poietic death without overlapping with the gastrointestinal region is narrower in most animals than in the mouse.

When considering the immunosuppressive properties of X-ray, it is useful to compare it with the other immunosuppressive agents. An operational classi-fication of such agents has been proposed based on when the immune re-sponse is most sensitive to a given modality (Makinodan et al., 1970).

Class I agents are most effective in suppressing an immune response when given before the antigenic stimulus and are relatively ineffective when given after. The very early processes of the immune response on which these agents are assumed to act include antigen processing and early "information" transfer.

Class II agents are most effective as immunosuppressants when given a day or two after the antigenic stimulus. The period of maximal sensitivity may last a day or two. In general, the cellular proliferation and differentiation of the immune response are more sensitive than other stages of the immune response to the action of these compounds. Furthermore, they are quite in-effective as immunosuppressants when given before the antigen; indeed, some of the agents may enhance the immune response under these conditions. The majority of immunosuppressive drugs such as antimetabolites are in this class.

Class III agents comprise the smallest group of drugs. They appear to be immunosuppressants whether applied solely before the antigenic stimulus or solely after the stimulus, and thus appear to possess the properties of both class I and class II agents.

The immunosuppressive properties of X-ray have been well studied, and it is evident that it is primarily effective only when applied just before the antigenic stimulus, and therefore it has been considered a class I agent (Makinodan et al., 1970). Marrow transplantation has usually been performed several hours to 24 hr after irradiation. In rodent species there is some evi-dence that 24 hr is optimal. However, this has not been entirely well studied with variables of cell dose and time interval (van Bekkum and deVries, 1967). The number of bone marrow takes and length of persistence (time to reversal of chimeric state) are quite clearly related to X-ray dose (Santos *et al.*, 1958). In general, one has to employ doses well into the supralethal range in order to effect long-lasting or permanent chimerism. Occasionally, long-lasting mixed chimerism occurs in rodent chimeras. The majority of animals, however, are complete chimeras or eventually reject donor-type cells. Furthermore, the rate of conversion of mixed chimeras to total reversal appears to be directly proportional to the degree of histoincompatibility between host and donor (i.e., histocompatible cells will enjoy a longer chimeric state for a given dose of X-ray) (van Bekkum and deVries, 1967).

In general, successful bone marrow transplantation following supralethal doses of X-ray is accomplished with smaller numbers of syngeneic then allogeneic cells. The number of parental cells, for instance, required to protect lethally irradiated F_1 hybrid mice is equal to the number of syngeneic cells. In the reverse combination, many more cells are required (van Bekkum and Vos, 1957), as is the case with allogeneic or xenogeneic bone marrow cells. One exception to this general pattern of parent strain bone marrow efficacy has been discovered. When C57BL/6 marrow is used to restore F_1 hybrids, up to ten times as many cells are required as in the case of marrow from the other parent strain (McCulloch and Till, 1961; Popp, 1961, Popp *et al.*, 1964; Lotzova and Cudkowicz, 1971). The basis of this exceptional difference in mice was not known until recently but will be elucidated later under a description of GVH disease. Thus, there are many reasons (some to be elucidated in the next section) to support the belief that even a high dose of total-body irradiation does not completely suppress the capacity of the recipient to react against foreign antigens and that a factor of 5 to 15 between the recolonizing capacity of syngeneic as opposed to allogeneic hematopoietic cells may exist.

Treatment with syngeneic bone marrow is generally successful in preventing death at all X-ray doses up to those which are followed by the intestinal syndrome. Several investigators have reported the existence of a lower limit of irradiation dose following which transplantation of allogeneic or xenogeneic bone marrow and subsequent recovery can be obtained (Gengozian and Makinodan, 1957; Trentin, 1956). They observed, moreover, that in the midlethal dose region the injection of allogeneic or xenogeneic bone marrow is ineffective and in some cases even harmful. The term *midlethal dose effect* (MLD effect) has been proposed only to designate the fact that the administration of foreign bone marrow causes an increased death rate when compared with irradiated controls, rather than to apply to all cases where foreign bone marrow is merely ineffective. The basis of this effect is a situation wherein the recipient animal retains enough immune competence to reject the foreign graft but not enough hematopoietic potential to completely repair itself. The increased death rate would seem to be related to nonspecific effects of the rejection process upon hematopoietic tissue. This phenomenon has only been observed in mice and then only in a situation of a few strain combinations (Uphoff, 1963) and appears to be the exception rather than the rule even in mice. Although the experiment has not been done, one would predict that on the basis of the above that the LD_{50} dose of X-irradiation would be less in mice presensitized to a given donor when that donor was used for marrow donation after exposure to X-irradiation. The discovery of this effect suggests that caution must be exercised in clinical cases of accidental whole-body irradiation, where the exact exposure may not accurately be known.

The alkylating agent, CY, is a powerful immunosuppressant in animals and man (Santos et al., 1970b; Makinodan et al., 1970). In single doses, CY suppresses immune responses when given before or after the antigenic stimulus and is therefore called a class III agent. However, the greatest effect is seen when CY is administered 24-48 hr after the antigenic stimulus. Nevertheless, the drug when given before the antigenic stimulus in rodents has a high therapeutic ratio for immunosuppression. In man, the drug administered as single or multiple injections at several different dose levels was not reproducibly immunosuppressive if given solely before the antigenic stimulus (Vi or *Pasteurella tularensis* vaccine) but had considerable effect when given a day or two after it (Santos et al., 1970b).

In mice, a pure "bone marrow" death cannot be produced with CY. As one increases the dose of drug into the lethal range, the first deaths seen are rather acute and are probably related to CNS effects (Santos, unpublished observations). Nevertheless, the drug is quite immunosuppressive and permits engraftment of lymphohematopoietic histoincompatible allogeneic cells at sublethal doses with the establishment of a long-term chimeric state (Santos and Owens, 1969).

When Balb/c $\times$ DBA/2 (CD2F$_1$) mice were given graded single doses of CY followed in 24 hr by 20 $\times$ 10^6 C57BL/6 or C3Hanf $\times$ C57BL/6 (C3BF$_1$) marrow, the number of animals shown to be chimeras and the time of persistence of the chimeric state were shown to be related to the dose of drug administered. Essentially all animals given 300-400 mg/kg of CY were shown to be chimeras at 1 year. Such animals retained donor-type skin, and no case of split tolerance was observed (Santos and Owens, 1969). GVH disease was seen in these animals and did not appear to differ from that seen following X-ray (Owens and Santos, 1968; Santos and Owens, 1969; Sandberg et al., 1971). Subsequent analyses of animals as noted previously reveal that the majority of mice are mixed chimeras (host and donor lymphohematopoietic cells are present) (Owens, personal communication).

In an attempt to quantitate the degrees of "take" of H-2 incompatible spleen cells in mice pretreated with CY, a system of adoptive transfer of antibody formation was employed. A linear $\log_2$ relation exists between antibody titer (anti-sheep erythrocyte agglutinin) and the number of viable nucleated syngeneic (Santos and Owens, 1966) or allogeneic (Santos, 1966b) cells transferred to CY pretreated mice. In the following experiments to be described, CD2F$_1$ mice were given graded doses of CY intraperitoneally. Four hours later, they were given sheep red blood cells (SRBC) alone or together with 16×10^6 C56BL/6 or CD2F$_1$ spleen cells. Agglutinin titers were determined 5 days later. The results are depicted in Fig. 2. Mice given 100 mg/kg or more of CY failed to respond serologically to SRBC. This was also true of the other strains used as recipients in further experiments. There was no effect of CY dose on the subsequent function of syngeneic cells. With increasing doses of CY up to 250 mg/kg, however, there was progressively greater function of the allogeneic cells. Below 250 mg/kg of CY, it would appear that the host, although unable to show a serological response to SRBC, is able to reject allogeneic spleen cells. Above 250 mg/kg of CY, a plateau is noted, suggesting "complete" suppression of the host vs. graft reaction in this system.

Table II contains data from experiments performed in an identical manner using CD2F$_1$, B6D2F$_1$, or C3B6F$_1$ recipients. Increasing doses of CY did not affect the function of syngeneic or parental cells, but did affect the function of allogeneic cells in a way quite similar to that illustrated in Fig. 2.

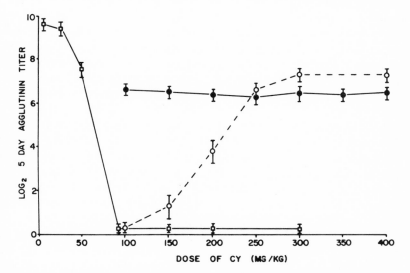

Figure 2. Effect of CY dose on antibody production by spleen cells transferred to CD2F$_1$ mice. □, CY only; ●, CY + 16×10^6 CD2F$_1$ spleen cells; ○, CY + 16×10^6 C3BF$_1$ spleen cells. Ten to twenty animals per point. Vertical bars represent ±SE. All animals given 1 ml of 1% SRBC 4 hr after CY.

Table II. Effect of CY Dose on Antibody Production by Adoptively Transferred Spleen Cells

Host	(mg/kg)	Mean 5-day $\log_2$ titer $\pm$ 1 SE after transfer of 16×10^6 spleen cells from various donors[a]					
		CD2F$_1$	DBA/2	BALB/c	C3B6F$_1$	C57BL/6	B6D2F$_1$
CD2F$_1$	100	6.60 ± 0.21	6.22 ± 0.35	6.80 ± 0.31	1.00 ± 0.35		
CD2F$_1$	150	6.50 ± 0.20	6.02 ± 0.46	6.00 ± 0.26	1.30 ± 0.40		
CD2F$_1$	200	6.40 ± 0.22	6.80 ± 0.15	6.20 ± 0.30	3.00 ± 0.40		
CD2F$_1$	250	6.30 ± 0.31	6.00 ± 0.24	6.90 ± 0.25	6.60 ± 0.31		
CD2F$_1$	300	6.45 ± 0.24	6.20 ± 0.26	6.70 ± 0.32	7.10 ± 0.29		
CD2F$_1$	350	6.40 ± 0.25			7.00 ± 0.21		
CD2F$_1$	400	6.50 ± 0.26	6.50 ± 0.34	7.00 ± 0.25	7.00 ± 0.26		
B6D2F$_1$	100		6.10 ± 0.40			6.20 ± 0.22	4.60 ± 0.23
B6D2F$_1$	200		6.20 ± 0.23			5.80 ± 0.26	4.80 ± 0.27
B6D2F$_1$	300		6.80 ± 0.35			6.70 ± 0.15	4.42 ± 0.31
B6D2F$_1$	400		6.20 ± 0.25			6.00 ± 0.20	4.52 ± 0.35
C3B6F$_1$	100				5.50 ± 0.15	6.22 ± 0.24	
C3B6F$_1$	200				5.40 ± 0.46	7.00 ± 0.42	
C3B6F$_1$	300				5.50 ± 0.15	7.22 ± 0.21	
C3B6F$_1$	400				5.60 ± 0.26	7.00 ± 0.36	

[a]Spleen cells transferred intravenously together with 1 ml of 1% SRBC intraperitoneally 4 hr after CY to the host. Ten to twenty mice were used for each mean.

Above 250 mg/kg of CY, the titers observed with allogeneic cells, and also with parental cells in the case of the B6D2F$_1$ and CD2F$_1$ recipients, were always higher than those seen after syngeneic transfer. This phenomenon of "allogeneic enhancement" has been documented and commented upon (Santos, 1966b). It probably represents an adjuvant effect of GVH disease, since it did not occur in situations where GVH disease could not occur (i.e., hybrid cells transferred to the parent) (Santos, unpublished observations).

It is instructive to compare the above studies with those of Celada and Carter (1962), who studied agglutinin production by allogeneic spleen cells in X-rayed recipient mice. They noted that increasing the dose of X-ray (as high as 900 r) to the host resulted in progressively higher antibody titers by the transferred cells. No "plateau" was observed, and "allogeneic enhancement" was not seen. It should be noted that 900 r represents a supralethal dose of X-ray and that the high dose of CY employed in the studies cited above is not a lethal dose. For these reasons and those to be developed in the following paragraphs, it is likely that CY has a higher therapeutic ratio for immuno-suppression than does X-ray and, furthermore, that residual host reactivity exists even at supralethal doses of X-ray.

Experiments in the rat have indicated that CY may produce a bone marrow type of death that can be reversed by the infusion of syngeneic or allogeneic marrow (Santos and Owens, 1968a). As in the mouse, the number of animals made chimeric and the time of persistence of chimerism are related to the dose of CY administered. Furthermore, no midlethal dose effect is seen (Santos and Owens, 1968a). The range of doses of CY required to produce chimerism with AgB-incompatible cells in essentially 100% of the animals is narrow. Thus, 200 mg/kg does not, but 225-250 mg/kg does permit chimerism in essentially 100% of the animals so treated. Doses of CY exceeding 250 mg/kg in the rat strain employed in these studies produced a nonmarrow type of death (i.e., syngeneic marrow afforded no protection). In contrast to mixed chimerism observed in mice, rats that received 225 mg/kg of CY followed in 24 hr by AgB-incompatible cells were complete chimeras as best as could be determined by typing bone marrow and peripheral blood cells with cytotoxic isoantisera. These animals accepted donor-type skin (survival for greater than 1 year) but promptly rejected third-party skin allografts (Santos and Owens, 1968a).

As stated above, CY did not suppress antibody formation in man when large but nonlethal doses of drug were administered prior to immunization. It was demonstrated, however, that specific nonreactivity to a given antigen could be induced in man by injecting the antigen in question a day or two before a course of CY (Santos et al., 1970b). It was also shown that CY could be employed to induce specific tolerance in mice to cells of another histoincompatible strain (Santos et al., 1970b; Santos and Owens, 1968b). In this system, the survival and function of spleen cell grafts were measured by the amount of antibody they produced. Recipient mice were given 100 mg/kg of CY. At this dose, they failed to develop antibody after the injection of SRBC. They retained the immunological capability of rejecting the spleen cells from a histoincompatible mouse, however, and the injection of such spleen cells together with SRBC produced no antibody (see Fig. 2). If, however, spleen cells from one strain of mice were injected intravenously 24 hr before CY, the mice would subsequently accept spleen cells from the strain that donated the first injection of spleen cells but not from other strains of mice. To produce this tolerant state, optimal conditions were met for both the route of administration and time of administration when donor spleen cells were given intravenously 24 hr before CY (Santos and Owens, 1968b). An example of a typical experiment is given in Table III. It was subsequently shown that marrow grafts could be obtained in dogs employing this principle (Storb et al., 1969). Dogs were given an infusion of blood from a female donor. Twenty-four hours later, they were given 100 mg/kg of CY (LD_{100}). Twenty-four hours after CY, marrow was transplanted from the donor. This procedure yielded successful transplants, as demonstrated by karyotype analysis in a number of dogs. It is of interest, however, that these dogs remained stable

Table III. Effect of Dose of CY With and Without Donor Type Preimmunization on the Function of Adoptively Transferred Allogeneic Spleen Cells

Pretreatment	Dose of CY (mg/kg)	Mean $\log_2$ titer[a] $\pm$ 1 SE
None	100	0.30 ± 0.15
	150	1.30 ± 0.39
	200	3.80 ± 0.46
	250	6.60 ± 0.21
	300	7.30 ± 0.15
	400	7.30 ± 0.26
16×10^6 cells[b]	100	6.40 ± 0.15
	150	7.70 ± 0.24
	200	7.80 ± 0.42
	300	7.60 ± 0.21

[a]Agglutinin titer produced by 16×10^6 C57BL/6 preimmunized nucleated spleen cells transferred to $CD2F_1$ hosts together with SRBC 4 hr after various doses of CY.

[b]C57BL/6 nucleated spleen cells injected nitravenously 24 hr before CY.

mixed chimeras (both host and donor lymphohematopoietic cells). Marrow grafts were subsequently obtained in man (Bach *et al.*, 1968; Santos *et al.*, 1970*b*, 1971*a*; Graw *et al.*, 1971) and the monkey (Storb *et al.*, 1970*b*) using this principle.

A possible mechanism for the specificity of "drug-induced immunological tolerance" is that the first injection of antigen given just before CY "selects" the immunocompetent cells responsive to it and causes them to undergo proliferation and differentiation. These cells are selectively killed because they are more sensitive to the cytotoxic action of CY than are unstimulated immunocompetent cells. When the same antigen is given later, there are no cells left that are able to respond to it, but other antigens can arouse an immune response in appropriate surviving cells.

In man, the practice has been to infuse donor antigen in the form of 1 unit of whole blood 24 hr prior to the administration of CY. The drug has been given as 45-60 mg/kg on each of 4 successive days. Marrow is infused 24 hr after the last dose of drug. Serious cardiac toxicity in the form of hemorrhagic carditis has been seen at total doses of 240 mg/kg and above in at least three instances (Santos *et al.*, 1971*a*; Thomas, personal communication; Bortin, personal communication). This has also been observed in the monkey (Storb *et al.*, 1970*b*). Although carditis has not been seen at a total dose of 180 mg/kg of (45 mg/kg × 4) (Graw *et al.*, 1971), that dose does not appear to provide sufficient immunosuppression to permit the establishment of complete chimerism (see discussion of treatment of malignancy above). The optimal dose would seem to be somewhere between a total dose of 180 mg/kg and 240 mg/kg, a situation that by chance happens to be what pertains in the rat, as discussed above. Apart from potential cardiac toxicity, patients given a total dose of 240 mg/kg tend to retain fluid for a brief period following CY treatment (Santos *et al.*, 1971*a*). This complication, however, is readily manageable, but its mechanism is unexplained. One patient who received a total of 240 mg/kg and subsequently oral CY to control GVH disease developed an interstitial pneumonitis of unknown etiology. This has also recently been observed in a patient with lymphosarcoma who received more conventional (no transplant) doses of the drug (Mullins *et al.*, in preparation). It is thought to be a rare form of toxicity to the drug not unlike that seen occasionally with busulfan (Oliner *et al.*, 1961) or MTX (Clarysse *et al.*, 1969). The pulmonary condition responded in both patients to the administration of prednisone.

In some, if not the majority of cases of aplastic anemia with pancytopenia, there is either a deficiency of or a defect in H cells without an associated loss of function of the lymphoid system. Accordingly, immunosuppression may be required if an allogeneic marrow graft is to be successful.

Busulfan (myleran) is not immunosuppressive in the rat (Santos, 1966*a*), and dimethyl myleran is not immunosuppressive in the mouse (Floersheim and

Ruszkiewicz, 1969). Rats given lethal doses of busulfan (Santos, 1966a) and mice given lethal doses of dimethyl myleran (Floersheim and Ruszkiewicz, 1969) can be protected from lethal drug toxicity with syngeneic but not allogeneic marrow grafts. Allogeneic grafts fail because these myelosuppressed animals retain sufficient immunological reactivity to reject allogeneic cells. These animal systems provide models for clinical cases of aplastic anemia.

Floersheim and Ruszkiewicz (1969) gave mice seven daily subcutaneous injections of ALS ending 5 days before the administration of lethal doses of dimethyl myleran and the infusion of allogeneic marrow or spleen cells. Protection from dimethyl myleran toxicity was noted; however, additional deaths were seen due to GVH disease. As noted previously, Amiel et al. (1970) and Rogentine et al. (1970) demonstrated that marrow takes were possible in some clinical cases of aplastic anemia when ALG was employed for immuno-suppression. In view of the GVH reaction seen in the mouse system described above, it is perhaps surprising that Amiel et al. (1970) did not observe GVH in their clinical cases. The last injection of ALG in the latter situation was given 24 hr prior to transplantation, and perhaps sufficient ALG was present in the circulation to directly immunosuppress donor lymphocytes in the marrow infusion.

Table IV summarizes the results of experiments performed in inbred rats given syngeneic or allogeneic histocompatible or allogeneic histoincompatible marrow grafts following lethal doses of busulfan alone or with CY. It is clear that only syngeneic marrow successfully protects against busulfan toxicity. However, the additional administration of CY allows the engraftment of allo-geneic marrow with protection from drug toxicity. Survival with allogeneic

Table IV. Marrow Transplants in Drug-Treated Lewis Rats

Donor[a]	Survival at 28 days	
	BU	BU + CY
Lewis	10/10	10/10
F344	0/10	10/10
Buf	0/10	6/10
WF	0/10	8/10
ACI	0/10	9/10
BN	0/10	7/10
No cells	0/10	0/10

[a] Lewis rats given 30 mg/kg of busulfan (BU) or 30 mg/kg of BU + 100 mg/kg of CY 24 hr before 64×10^6 marrow cells.

histoincompatible marrow is not 100% because of deaths due to GVH disease. Most recently, Thomas *et al.* (1971*c*) were able to demonstrate that CY could be employed successfully for allogeneic marrow transplantation in clinical aplastic anemia. These workers employed CY as outlined by Santos *et al.* (1971*a*) in a female with a relatively recent onset of aplasia. The marrow donor was a histocompatible brother, and proof of engraftment was shown by karyotype analysis of the peripheral blood and marrow.

It is most encouraging that the pertinence and usefulness of the animal models described above have so soon been verified in the clinic.

PROBLEMS RELATED TO THE PRESENSITIZED STATE

Special problems of immunosuppression arise when the individual has been presensitized to the transplantation antigens of the donor. In animals, the injection of relatively few donor-type cells several days prior to transplantation will presensitize the recipient against xenogeneic (Santos *et al.*, 1959) or allogeneic histoincompatible or allogeneic histocompatible grafts (i.e., H-2 or DL-A identical grafts) (Santos *et al.*, 1971*b*; Storb *et al.*, 1970*c*, 1971); Van Putten *et al.*, 1967). Under these conditions in the dog, the rejection of allogeneic marrow may be somewhat delayed and there may be initial evidence of engraftment with subsequent failure of the graft. This latter phenomenon is important to remember when attempting to understand the mechanism of transient graft function in clinical trials. Of perhaps greater importance is the observation that cells from third-party donors (unrelated to host and donor) may be capable of sensitizing animals to allogeneic histoincompatible as well as to allogeneic histocompatible grafts (Santos *et al.*, 1971*b*; Storb *et al.*, 1971). In many of these situations, particularly where sensitization to minor transplantation antigens is involved, measurable cytotoxic antibody is absent in the sera (Santos *et al.*, 1971*b*; Storb *et al.*, 1970*c*).

These studies have practical significance in that transfusions, particularly from family members of potential donors, should be avoided or at least minimized in patients who are to be candidates for marrow transplantation. On the other hand, HL-A histocompatible siblings provide the best donors of platelets for the patient who has received multiple transfusions (Yankee *et al.*, 1969). Thus the clinician is presented with a difficult dilemma that must be resolved in each individual case.

At present, there is no evidence that the presensitized state can be eliminated; however, it is hoped that newer efforts, particularly with ALS, will provide the necessary information for practical solutions to this problem.

GVH DISEASE

GVH disease has been encountered in several situations in which individuals have been unable to defend themselves against grafts of immunologically competent allogeneic cells either because of immunoincompetence produced by disease states (Bergsma and Good, 1967) or because of immunosuppressive treatment (van Bekkum and deVries, 1967). The clinical and pathological aspects of this disease in animals and man have been extensively reviewed elsewhere (van Bekkum and deVries, 1967). It is presently clear that the pathogenesis of GVH disease is not as simple as might have originally been conceived. Thus the disease is not created simply because a lymphocyte (thought to be a T lymphocyte) causes a direct destruction of a host target cell. One must take into consideration the recent observations that sensitized lymphocytes will liberate a variety of pharmacologically active factors when presented with appropriate antigen (Lawrence and Valentine, 1970). It is probable that these substances play a role in the pathogenesis of the disease. Hematopoiesis may be nonspecifically suppressed by GVH disease, and Sensenbrenner and Santos (1970) have shown that the addition of donor type lymph node cells will decrease the number of hematopoietic colonies in the spleen of drug-treated mice given allogeneic marrow cells. The data reported by these workers suggest that the F_1 effect noted previously (wherein parental marrow appears to function poorly in the hybrid mouse) is due to the generation of nonspecific toxic effects elicited by T lymphocytes (in the donor marrow) as they react to host antigens. It is hoped that further understanding of these phenomena will suggest additional means of ameliorating the severity of GVH disease.

Some success in reducing the severity of GVH disease in animals has been achieved with the use of CY (van Bekkum and deVries, 1967; Owens and Santos, 1971), methotrexate (van Bekkum and deVries, 1967; Storb et al., 1970a), and ALS (Ledney, 1969) given immediately after transplantation. In addition, fractionation of marrow (in order to remove T lymphocytes) has been shown to be effective (Dicke et al., 1969).

In man, there have not been enough clinical trials to indicate which of the above methods might be employed to successfully control severe GVH disease. The results of the administration of CY and methotrexate after transplantation of HL-A matched sibling transplants, however, has been encouraging. Of 16 such marrow transplants, performed by the groups at Johns Hopkins University (Santos et al., 1971a), the University of Washington (Thomas et al., 1971b), and The National Cancer Institute (Graw et al., 1971), where there was evidence of engraftment, mild (transient skin rash) or no GVH disease was seen in six patients. Moderately severe GVH disease with definite skin involvement and occasional liver function abnormalities was seen in five.

Severe GVH disease that led to death occurred in five. It is of interest that three of the five patients with severe GVH disease either did not receive post-transplant immunosuppressive treatment or were given unirradiated lymphocytes contaminating platelet infusions (a situation known to increase the severity of GVH disease in animals).

One of the most promising approaches to the control of GVH disease has been suggested by the observation that donor cell populations eventually develop "tolerance" to host antigens after GVH disease (Santos, 1967a; Santos and Owens, 1969; Santos et al., 1970c). Hellström et al. (1970) demonstrated with the aid of the colony inhibition test that "tolerance" of donor cells to the host in long-term dog chimeras occurred because of the production of a serum enhancing or blocking factor that effectively and specifically abrogates cell-mediated immunity against host antigens. Field et al. (1967) had reported previously that refractoriness to GVH disease could be transferred to F_1 rats employing serum from animals that had recovered from GVH disease.

In addition, Voisin et al. (1968) were able to prepare "enhancing" sera that under certain conditions were able to effectively blunt the severity of GVH disease. Most recently, Buckley et al. (1971) reported that enhancing factor could be demonstrated in the sera of a previously pregnant woman that successfully prevented fatal GVH disease in two histoincompatible marrow transplants to an infant with lymphopenic agammaglobulinemia. It is hoped that further investigation with enhancing factor (probably a 7S-immunoglobulin) will lead to a highly specific and nontoxic means of controlling GVH disease.

CONCLUSIONS

The rationale, potential, and some of the problems associated with the application of marrow grafts in human disease have been outlined. There have been a few notable and dramatic successes, but overall the majority of clinical trials have met with failure. Nevertheless, the information gained in the theoretical and practical sense does suggest some optimism for the future. Continued animal and clinical research on the nature and control of GVH disease, the prevention and elimination of the presensitized state, and the supportive care of individuals during periods of aplasia hopefully will justify the optimism.

REFERENCES

Aldrich, R. A., Steinberg, A. C., and Campbell, D. C., 1954. Pedigree demonstrating a sex-linked recessive condition characterized by draining ears, eczematoid dermatitis and bloody diarrhea. *Pediatrics* 13:133.

Amato, D., Bergsagel, D. E., Clarysse, A. M., Cowan, D. H., Iscoue, N. N., McCulloch, E. A., Miller, R. G., Phillips, R. A., Ragab, A. H., and Senn, J. S., 1971. Review of bone marrow transplants at the Ontario Cancer Institute. *Transplant. Proc.* 3:397.

Amiel, J. F., Mathé, G., Schwarzenberg, L., Schneider, M., Choay, J., Trolard, P., Hayat, M., Schlumberger, J. R., and Jasmin, C., 1970. Les greffes de moelle osseuse allogénique après conditionnement par le seul sérum antilymphocytaire dans les états d'aplasie médullaire. *Presse Med.* 78:1727.

August, C. S., Rosen, F. S., Filler, R. M., Janeway, C. A., Markowski, B., and Kay, H. E. M., 1968. Implantation of a fetal thymus restoring immunological competence in a patient with thymic aplasia (DiGeorge's syndrome). *Lancet* 2:1210.

Bach, F. H., 1970. Transplantation: Pairing of donor and recipient. *Science* 168:1170.

Bach, F. H., Joo, P., Albertini, R. J., Anderson, J. L., and Borton, M. M., 1968. Bone marrow transplantation in a patient with Wiskott-Aldrich syndrome. *Lancet* 2:1364.

Barnes, D. W. H., and Loutit, J. F., 1957. Treatment of murine leukaemia with X-rays and homologous bone marrow. II. *Brit. J. Haematol.* 3:241.

Barnes, D. W. H., Corp, M. J., Loutit, J. F., and Neal, F. F., 1956. Treatment of murine leukaemia with X-rays and homologous bone marrow. *Brit. Med. J.* 2:626.

Beilby, J. O. W., Cade, I, S., Jellife, A. M., Parkin, D. M., and Stewart, J. W., 1960. Prolonged survival of a bone marrow graft resulting in a blood-group chimera. *Brit. Med. J.* 1:96.

Bergsma, D., and Good, R. A., eds., 1967. *Immunologic Deficiency Diseases in Man,* The National Foundation–March of Dimes, New York, pp. 1–473.

Bernstein, S. E., 1970. Tissue transplantation as an analytic and therapeutic tool in hereditary anemias. *Am. J. Surg.* 119:448.

Boranić, M., 1968. Transient graft versus host reaction in the treatment of leukemia in mice. *J. Natl. Cancer Inst.* 41:421.

Bortin, M., 1970. A compendium of reported human bone marrow transplants. *Transplantation* 9:571.

Boyse, E. A., Lance, E. M., Carswell, E. A., Cooper, S., and Old, L. J., 1971. Rejection of skin allografts by radiation chimeras: Selective gene action in the specification of cell surface structure. *Nature* 227:901.

Brockman, W. W., Carter, W. A., Li, H. L., Reusser, F., and Nichol, F. R., 1971. The streptovaricins inhibit RNA dependent DNA polymerase present in an oncogenic RNA virus. *Nature* 230:249.

Buckley, R. H., Lucas, Z. J., Hattler, B. G., Jr., Zmijewski, C. M., and Amos, D. B., 1968. Defective cellular immunity associated with chronic mucocutaneous moniliasis and recurrent staphylococcal botryomycosis: Immunological reconstitution by allogeneic bone marrow. *Clin. Exptl. Immunol.* 3:153.

Buckley, R. H., Schiff, R. I., and Amos, B. D., 1971. Human enhancing antibodies: *In vitro* studies. *Fed. Proc.* 30:936.

Buckner, C. D., Epstein, R. B., Rudolph, R. H., Clift, R. A., Storb, R., and Thomas, E. D., 1970. Allogeneic marrow engraftment following whole body irradiation in a patient with leukemia. *Blood* 35:741.

Canales, L., Louro, J. M., Middlemas, R. O., and South, M. A., 1969. Immunological observations in chronic mucocutaneous candidiasis. *Lancet* 2:567.

Celada, F., and Carter, R. R., 1962. The radiosensitive nature of homograft-rejecting and agglutinin-forming capacities of isolated spleen cells. *J. Immunol.* 89:161.

Chilgren, R. S., Meuwissen, H. J., Quie, P. G., and Hong, R., 1967. Chronic mucocutaneous candidiasis, deficiency of delayed hypersensitivity and selective local antibody defect. *Lancet* 2:688.

Chilgren, R. S., Meuwissen, H. J., Quie, P. G., Good, R. A., and Hong, R., 1969. The cellular immune defect in chronic mucocutaneous candidiasis. *Lancet* 1:1286.

Clarysse, A. M., Cathey, W. J., Cartwright, G. E., and Wintrobe, M. M., 1969. Pulmonary disease complicating intermittent therapy with methotrexate. *J.A.M.A.* 209:1861.

Cleveland, W. W., Fogel, B. J., Brown, W. T., and Kay, H. E. M., 1968. Fetal thymic transplant in a case of DiGeorge's syndrome. *Lancet* 2:1211.

Congdon, C. C., 1970. Cooperative group on bone marrow transplantation in man: Report of work sessions held June 16-17, at Hôpital Paul-Brousse, Villejuif, France. *Exptl. Hematol.* 20:97.

Cooper, M. D., Perey, D. Y., Peterson, R. D. A., Gabrielsen, A. E., and Good, R. A., 1967. The two-component concept of the lymphoid system. In Bergsma, D., and Good, R. A., eds., *Immunologic Deficiency Diseases in Man,* The National Foundation-March of Dimes, New York, pp. 7-12.

Cooper, M. D., Chase, H. P., Lowman, J. T., Krivit, W., and Good, R. A., 1968. Wiskott-Aldrich syndrome: An immunologic deficiency disease involving the afferent limb of immunity. *Am. J. Med.* 44:499.

DeKoning, J., Dooren, L. J., van Bekkum, D. W., van Rood, J. J., Dieke, K. A., and Radl, J., 1969. Transplantation of bone marrow cells and fetal thymus in an infant with lymphopenic immunological deficiency. *Lancet* 1:1223.

deVaal, O. M., and Seynhaeve, V., 1959. Reticular dysgenesia. *Lancet* 2:1123.

deVries, M. J., and Vos, O., 1958. Treatment of mouse lymphosarcoma by total-body X-irradiation and by injection of bone marrow and lymph node cells. *J. Natl. Cancer Inst.* 21:1117.

deVries, M. J., and Vos, O., 1960. Treatment of mouse lymphosarcoma by total-body irradiation and administration of bone marrow and lymph node cells. The effect of isologous lymph node cells. *Acta Unio Internat. Contra Cancrum* 16:1165.

Dicke, K. A., Tridente, G., and van Bekkum, D. W., 1969. The selective elimination of immunologically competent cells from bone marrow and lymphocyte cell mixtures. III. *In vitro* test for detection of immunocompetent cells in fractionated mouse spleen cell suspensions and primate bone marrow suspensions. *Transplantation* 8:422.

DiGeorge, A. M., 1967. Congenital absence of the thymus and its immunologic consequences: Concurrence with congenital hypoparathyroidism. In Bergsma, D., and Good, R. A., eds., *Immunologic Deficiency Diseases in Man,* The National Foundation-March of Dimes, New York, pp. 116-121.

Dooren, L. J., deVries, M. J., van Bekkum, D. W., Cleton, F. J., and DeKoning, J., 1968. Sex-linked thymic epithelial hypoplasia in two siblings. *J. Pediat.* 72:51.

Douglas, S. D., and Fudenberg, H. H., 1969. Graft versus host reaction in Wiskott-Aldrich syndrome: Antemortem diagnosis of human GVH in an immunologic deficiency disease. *Vox Sang* 16:172.

Epstein, R. B., Graham, T. C., Storb, R., and Thomas, E. D., 1971. Studies of marrow transplantation, chemotherapy and cross circulation in canine lymphosarcoma. *Blood* 37:349.

Fefer, A., 1970. Immunotherapy of primary Moloney sarcoma virus-induced tumors. *Internat. J. Cancer* 5:327.

Fialkow, P. J., Thomas, E. D., Bryant, J. I., and Neiman, P. E., 1971. Leukemic transformation of engrafted human marrow cells *in vivo. Lancet* 1:251.

Field, E. O., Cuchi, M. N., and Gibbs, J. E., 1967. The transfer of refractoriness to graft versus host disease in F_1 hybrid rats. *Transplantation* 5:241.

Floersheim, G. L., 1969. Treatment of Moloney lymphoma with lethal doses of dimethyl-myleran combined with injections of haemopoietic cells. *Lancet* 1:228.

Floersheim, G. L., and Ruszkiewicz, M., 1969. Bone marrow transplantation after anti-lymphocyte serum and lethal chemotherapy. *Nature* 222:854.

Gengozian, N., and Makinodan, T., 1957. Mortality of mice as affected by variation of X-ray dose and number of nucleated rat bone marrow cells injected. *Cancer Res.* 17:970.

Githens, J. H., Muschenheim, F., Fulginiti, V. A., Robinson, A., and Kay, H. E. M., 1969. Thymic alymphoplasia with XX/XY lymphoid chimerism secondary to probable maternal-fetal transfusion. *J. Pediat.* 75:87.

Gitlin, D., Vawter, G., and Craig, M. M., 1964. Thymic alymphoplasia and congenital aleukocytosis. *Pediatrics* 33:184.

Good, R. A., Peterson, R. D. A., Perey, D. Y., Finstad, J., and Cooper, M. D., 1967. In Bergsma, D., and Good, R. A., eds., *Immunologic Deficiency Diseases in Man,* The National Foundation-March of Dimes, New York, pp. 17-34.

Graw, R. G., Leventhal, B. G., Yankee, R. A., Rogentine, G. N., Whang-Peng, J., Herzig, G. P., Halterman, R. H., and Henderson, E. S., 1971. HL-A and mixed leukocyte culture matched allogeneic bone marrow transplantation in patients with acute leukemia. *Transplant. Proc.* 3:405.

Hathaway, W. E., Githens, J. K., Blackburn, W. R., *et al.*, 1965a. Aplastic anemia, histiocytosis and erythrodermia in immunologically deficient children: Probable human runt disease. *New Engl. J. Med.* 273:953.

Hathaway, W. E., Brangle, R. W., Nelson, T. L., *et al.*, 1965b. Aplastic anemia and a lymphocytosis in an infant with hypogammaglobulinemia: Graft versus host reaction? *J. Pediat.* 68:713.

Hathaway, W. E., Fulginiti, V. A., Pierce, C. W., Githens, J. H., Pearlman, D. S., Muschenheim, F., and Kempe, C. H., 1967. Graft versus host reaction following a single blood transfusion. *J.A.M.A.* 201:1015.

Heilmeyer, L., 1966. Die Atransferrinamien. *Acta Haematol.* 36:40.

Hellström, K. E., Hellström, I., and Brawn, J., 1969. Abrogation of cellular immunity to antigenically foreign mouse embryonic cells by a serum factor. *Nature* 224:914.

Hellström, I., Hellström, K. E., Storb, R., and Thomas, E. D., 1970. Colony inhibition of fibroblasts from chimeric dogs mediated by the dog's own lymphocytes and specifically abrogated by their serum. *Proc. Natl. Acad. Sci.* 66:65.

Hitzig, W. H., and Willi, H., 1961. Hereditare lymphoplasmocytare dysgenesie ("Alymphocytose mit Agammeglobulinamie"). *Schweiz. Med. Wschr.* 91:1625.

Hollcroft, J., Lorenz, E., Congdon, C. C., and Jacobson, L. O., 1953. Factors influencing the irradiation treatment of experimental lymphoid tumors. *Rev. Mex. Radiol.* 7:115.

Hong, R., Gatti, R. A., and Good, R. A., 1968. Hazard and potential benefits of blood transfusion in immunological deficiency. *Lancet* 2:388.

Hoyer, J. R., Cooper, M. D., Gabrielsen, A. E., and Good, R. A., 1967. Lymphopenic forms of congenital immunological deficiency: Clinical and pathological patterns. In Bergsma, D., and Good, R. A., eds., *Immunologic Deficiency Diseases in Man,* The National Foundation-March of Dimes, New York, pp. 91-103.

Imperato, P. J., Buckley, C. E., III, and Callaway, J. L., 1968. Candida granuloma. A clinical and immunology study. *Arch. Dermatol.* 97:139.

Jacobson, L. L., Marks, E. K., Simmons, E. L., Gaston, E. O., and Zirkle, R. E., 1949. Effect of spleen protection on mortality following X-irradiation. *J. Lab. Clin. Med.* 34:1538.

Jammet, H., Mathé, G. Pendic, B., Duplan, J. F., Maupin, B., Latarjet, R., Kalic, D., Schwartzenberg, L., Djukic, Z., and Vigne, J., 1959. Etude de six cas d'irradiation total aiguë accidentelle. *Rev. Franc. Etud. Clin. Biol.* 4:210.

Kadowaki, J., Thompson, R., Zuelzer, W. W., Wooley, P. V. J., Brough, A. J., and Gruber, P., 1965. XX/XY lymphoid chimerism in congenital immunological deficiency syndrome with thymic alymphoplasia. *Lancet* 2:1152.

Kay, H. E. M., 1970. States of immune deficiency (editorial). *Rev. Europ. Etud. Clin. Biol.* 15:249.

Klein, G., Klein, E., and Haughton, G., 1966. Variation of antigenic characteristics between different mouse lymphomas induced by the Moloney virus. *J. Natl. Cancer Inst.* 36:607.

Krantz, S. B., and Kao, V., 1967. Studies on red cell aplasia. I. Demonstration of a plasma inhibitor to heme synthesis and an antibody to erythroblast nuclei. *Proc. Natl. Acad. Sci.* 58:493.

Lance, E. M., Boyse, E. A., Carswell, B., and Cooper, S., 1971. Rejection of skin allografts by irradiation chimeras. *Transplant. Proc.* 3:864.

Lawrence, H. S., and Valentine, F. T., 1970. Transfer factor and other mediators of cellular immunity. *Am. J. Pathol.* 60:437.

Ledney, G. D., 1969. Antilymphocyte serum in the therapy and prevention of acute secondary disease in mice. *Transplantation* 8:127.

Levin, A. S., Spitler, L. E., Stites, D. P., and Fudenberg, H. H., 1970. Wiskott-Aldrich syndrome, a genetically determined cellular immunologic deficiency: Clinical and laboratory responses to therapy with transfer factor. *Proc. Natl. Acad. Sci.* 67:821.

Levy, R. N., Sawitsky, A., Florman, A. L., and Rubin, E., 1965. Fatal aplastic anemia after hepatitis. *New Engl. J. Med.* 273:1118.

Lotzova, E., and Cudkowicz, G., 1971. Rejection of parental marrow grafts by irradiated F_1 hybrid mice: Frequent occurrence in laboratory strains. *Fed. Proc.* 30:1451.

Makinodan, T., Santos, G. W., and Quinn, R. P., 1970. Immunosuppressive drugs. *Pharm. Rev.* 22:189.

Marmor, M. E., and Barnett, E. V., 1968. Cutaneous anergy without systemic disease. A syndrome associated with mucocutaneous fungal infection. *Am. J. Med.* 44:979.

Mathé, G., 1968. Bone marrow transplantation. In Rappaport, F. T., and Dausset, J., eds., *Human Transplantation,* Grune and Stratton, New York, pp. 284-303.

Mathé, G., Amiel, J. L., Schwarzenberg, L., Cattan, A., and Schneider, M., 1963. Hematopoietic chimera in man after allogeneic (homologous) bone marrow transplantation. Control of the secondary syndrome. *Brit. Med. J.* 2:1633.

Mayer, T. C., and Green, M. C., 1968. An experimental analysis of the pigment defect caused by mutations at the *W* and *Sl* loci in mice. *Develop. Biol.* 18:62.

McCulloch, E. A., and Till, J. E., 1963. Repression of colony-forming ability of C57BL hematopoietic cells transplanted into non-isologous hosts. *J. Cell. Comp. Physiol.* 61:301.

McCulloch, E. A., Siminovitch, L., and Till, J. E., 1964. Spleen colony formation in anemic mice of genotype W/W^v. *Science* 144:844.

McCulloch, E. A., Siminovitch, L., Till, J. E., Russell, E. S., and Bernstein, S. E., 1965. The cellular basis of the genetically determined hematopoietic defect in anemic mice of genotype Sl/Sl^d. *Blood* 26:399.

Mekori, T., and Phillips, R. A., 1969. The immune response in mice of genotypes W/W^v and Sl/Sl^d. *Proc. Soc. Exptl. Biol. Med.* 132:115.

Meuwissen, H. J., Gatti, R. A., Terasaki, P. I., Hong, R., and Good, R. A., 1969. Treatment of lymphopenic hypogammaglobulinemia and bone marrow aplasia by transplantation of allogeneic marrow. *New Engl. J. Med.* 281:691.

Meuwissen, H. J., Rodey, G., McArthur, J., Pabst, H., Gatti, R., Chilgren, R., Hong, R., Frommel, D., Coifman, R., and Good, R. A., 1971. Bone marrow transplantation: Therapeutic usefulness and complications. *Am. J. Med.,* in press.

Miller, G. G., and Phillips, R. A., 1969. Separation of cells by velocity sedimentation. *J. Cell. Physiol.* 73:191.

Miller, J. F. A. P., 1964. Effect of thymic ablation and replacement. In Good, R. A., and Gabrielsen, A. E., eds., *The Thymus in Immunology,* Harper and Row, New York, pp. 436-464.

Miller, M. E., and Schieken, R. M., 1967. Thymic dysplasia. A separable entity from "Swiss agammaglobulinemia." *Am. J. Med. Sci.* 253:741.

Möller, G., 1969. Antigen sensitive cells, *Transplant. Rev.* 1:1.

Mullins, G. M., Slavin, R. E., Lenhard, R. E., Eggleston, J. C., and Santos, G. W., in preparation. Pulmonary interstitial pneumonitis with fibrosis associated with cyclophosphamide therapy.

Oliner, H., Schwartz, R., Rubin, F., and Dameshek, W., 1961. Interstitial pulmonary fibrosis following busulfan therapy. *Am. J. Med.* 31:134.

Olson, G. B., South, M. A., and Good, R. A., 1967. Phytohemagglutinin unresponsiveness of lymphocytes from babies with congenital rubella. *Nature* 214:695.

Oppenheim, J. J., Blaese, R. M., and Waldman, T. A., 1970. Defective lymphocyte transformation and delayed hypersensitivity in Wiskott-Aldrich syndrome. *J. Immunol.* 104:835.

Owens, A. H., Jr., 1970. Effect of graft versus host disease on the course of L1210 leukemia. *Exptl. Hematol.* **20**:43.

Owens, A. H., Jr., and Santos, G. W., 1968. The induction of graft versus host disease in mice treated with cyclophosphamide. *J. Exptl. Med.* **128**:277.

Owens, A. H., Jr., and Santos, G. W., 1971. The effect of cytotoxic drugs on graft versus host disease in mice. *Transplantation* **11**:378.

Peters, J. T., 1945. Equine infectious anemia transmitted to man. *Ann. Int. Med.* **23**:271.

Phillips, M. E., and Thorbecke, G. J., 1966. Studies on the serum proteins of chimeras. I. Identification and study of the site of origin of donor type serum proteins in adult rat into mouse chimeras. *Internat. Arch. Allergy* **29**:553.

Pillow, R. P., Epstein, R. B., Buckner, C. D., Giblett, E. R., and Thomas, E. D., 1966. Treatment of bone marrow failure by isogeneic marrow infusion. *New Engl. J. Med.* 275.

Popp, R. A., 1961. Regression of grafted bone marrow in homologous irradiated mouse chimeras. *J. Natl. Cancer Inst.* **26**:629.

Popp, R. A., Cosgrove, G. E., and Popp, D. M., 1964. Relative ability of parental marrows to repopulate lethally irradiated F_1 hybrids. *Ann. N.Y. Acad. Sci.* **114**:538.

Rocklin, R. E., Chilgren, R. A., Hong, R., and David, J. R., 1970. Transfer of cellular hypersensitivity in chronic mucocutaneous candidiasis monitored *in vivo* and *in vitro. Cell. Immunol.* **1**:290.

Rogentine, G. N., Rosenberg, S., Merritt, C. B., Yankee, R. A., Leventhal, B. G., Graw, R. G., Greipp, G., Whang-Peng, J., and Fahey, J. L., 1970. Successful allogeneic bone marrow transplantation in aplastic anemia. Presented at the American Society of Hematology, Puerto Rico, December.

Russell, E. S., 1963. Problems and potentialities in the study of genic action in the mouse. In Burdette, W. J., ed., *Methodology in Mammalian Genetics,* Holden-Day, San Francisco, pp. 217-232.

Russell, E. S., Smith, L. J., and Lawson, F. A., 1956. Implantation of normal blood forming tissue in radiated genetically anemic hosts. *Science* **124**:1076.

Sandberg, J. S., Owens, A. H., Jr., and Santos, G. W., 1971. Clinical and pathological characteristics of graft versus host disease produced in cyclophosphamide-treated adult mice. *J. Natl. Cancer Inst.* **46**:151-160.

Santos, G. W., 1966*a*. Effect of syngeneic, allogeneic and parental marrow infusions in busulfan-injected rats, with a note concerning effects of busulfan on antibody production. *Exptl. Hematol.* **9**:61.

Santos, G. W., 1966*b*. Adoptive transfer of immunologically competent cells. III. Comparative ability of allogeneic and syngeneic cells to produce a primary antibody response in the cyclophosphamide pretreated mouse. *J. Immunol.* **97**:587.

Santos, G. W., 1967*a*. Marrow transplantation in cyclophosphamide treated rats: Early donor to host tolerance and long lived chimerism. *Exptl. Hematol.* **13**:36.

Santos, G. W., 1967*b*. Immunosuppressive drugs. I. *Fed. Proc.* **26**:907.

Santos, G. W., 1970. Effect of graft versus host disease on a spontaneous adenocarcinoma in mice. *Exptl. Hematol.* **20**:46.

Santos, G. W., and Owens, A. H., Jr., 1966. Adoptive transfer of immunologically competent cells. I. Quantitative studies of antibody formation by syngeneic spleen cells in the cyclophosphamide pretreated mouse. *Bull. Johns Hopkins Hosp.* **118**:109.

Santos, G. W., and Owens, A. H., Jr., 1968*a*. Syngeneic and allogeneic marrow transplants in the cyclophosphamide pretreated rat. In Dausset, J., Hamburger, J., and Mathé, G., eds., *Advances in Transplantation,* Munksgaard, Copenhagen, pp. 431-436.

Santos, G. W., and Owens, A. H., Jr., 1968*b*. Immunization and tolerance to lymphoid allografts in cyclophosphamide (CY) treated mice. *Fed. Proc.* **27**:506.

Santos, G. W., and Owens, A. H., Jr., 1969. Allogeneic marrow transplantation in cyclo-phosphamide-treated mice. *Transplant. Proc.* 1:44.
Santos, G. W., Cole, L. J., and Roan, P. L., 1958. Effect of X-ray dose on the protective action and persistence of rat bone marrow in irradiated penicillin treated mice. *Am. J. Physiol.* 194:23.
Santos, G. W., Cole, L. J., and Garver, R. M., 1959. Antigeneic stimuli for transplanta-tion immunity to rat bone marrow heterografts in lethally X-irradiated mice. *J. Immunol.* 83:66.
Santos, G. W., Garver, R. M., and Cole, L. J., 1960. Acceptance of rat and mouse lung grafts by radiation chimeras. *N. Natl. Cancer Inst.* 24:1367.
Santos, G. W., Sensenbrenner, L. L., Burke, P. J., Colvin, M., Owens, A. H., Jr., Bias, W., and Slavin, R., 1970a. Marrow transplants in man utilizing cyclophosphamide. Summary of Baltimore experience. *Exptl. Hematol.* 20:78.
Santos, G. W., Burke, P. J., Sensenbrenner, L. L., and Owens, A. H., Jr., 1970b. Ration-ale for the use of cyclophosphamide as immunosuppression for marrow transplants in man. In Bertelli, A., and Monaco, A. P., eds., *International Symposium on Pharmacologic Treatment in Organ and Tissue Transplantation, Milan, Italy, 1969,* Exerpta Medica Foundation, Amsterdam, pp. 24-31.
Santos, G. W., Sensenbrenner, L. L., Burke, P. J., Colvin, O. M., Owens, A. H., Jr., Bias, W. B., and Slavin, R. E., 1971a. Marrow transplantation in man following cyclo-phosphamide. *Transplant. Proc.* 3:400.
Santos, G. W., Sensenbrenner, L. L., and Owens, A. H., Jr., 1971b. Immunogenicity of non-H-2 antigens—sensitive assays. *Fed. Proc.* 30:1831.
Scott, J. L., Cartwright, G. E., and Wintrobe, M. M., 1959. Acquired aplastic anemia: An analysis of thirty-nine cases and review of the pertinent literature. *Medicine* 38:119.
Sensenbrenner, L. L., and Santos, G. W., 1970. Effect of syngeneic and allogeneic lymph node cells on spleen colony forming units. *Fed. Proc.* 29:785.
Shapiro, M., 1967. Familial autohemolytic anemia and runting syndrome with rho-specific antibody. *Transfusion* 7:281.
Simmons, R. L., Wolf, S. M., Chandler, J. G., and Nastuk, W. L., 1965. Effect of allogeneic bone marrow on lethally irradiated thymectomized mice. *Proc. Soc. Exptl. Biol. Med.* 120:81.
Smith, L. H., and Congdon, C. C., 1968. Biological effects of ionizing radiation. In Rapaport, F. T., and Dausset, J., eds., *Human Transplantation,* Grune and Stratton, New York, pp. 510-525.
Stewart, J. W., 1964. Haemopoietic chimera. *Brit. Med. J.* 1:304.
Storb, R., Epstein, R. B., Rudolph, R. H., and Thomas, E. D., 1969. Allogeneic canine marrow transplantation following cyclophosphamide transplantation, 7:378.
Storb, R., Epstein, R. B., Graham, T. C., and Thomas, E. C., 1970a. Methotrexate regimens for control of graft versus host disease in dogs with allogeneic marrow grafts. *Transplantation* 9:240.
Storb, R., Buckner, C. D., Dillingham, L. A., and Thomas, E. D., 1970b. Cyclophos-phamide regimens in Rhesus monkeys with and without marrow infusion. *Cancer Res.* 30:2195.
Storb, R., Epstein, R. B., Rudolph, R. H., and Thomas, E. D., 1970c. The effect of prior transfusions on marrow grafts between histocompatible canine siblings. *J. Immunol.* 105:627.
Storb, R., Rudolph, R. H., Graham, T. C., and Thomas, E. D., 1971. The influence of transfusions from unrelated donors upon marrow grafts between histocompatible canine siblings. *J. Immunol.* 107:409.
Thomas, E. D., Collins, J. A., Herman, E. C., Jr., and Ferrebee, J. W., 1962. Marrow transplants in lethally irradiated dogs given methotrexate. *Blood* 19:217.
Thomas, E. D., Rudolph, R. H., Fefer, A., Storb, R., Slichter, S., and Buckner, C. D., 1971a. Isogeneic marrow grafting in man. *Exptl. Hematol.,* in press.

Thomas, E. D., Buckner, C. D., Rudolph, R. H., Fefer, A., Storb, R., Neiman, P. E., Bryant, J. I., Chard, R. L., Clift, R. A., Epstein, R. B., Fialkow, P. J., Funk, D. D., Giblett, E. R., Lerner, K. G., Reynolds, F. A., and Slichter, S., 1971*b*. Allogeneic marrow grafting for hematologic malignancy HL-A matched donor-recipient sibling pairs. *Blood*, in press.

Thomas, E. D., Bryant, J. I., Buckner, C. D., Clift, R. A., Fefer, A., Fialkow, P. J., Funk, D. D., Neiman, P. E., Rudolph, R. H., Slichter, S. J., and Storb, R., 1971*c*. Allogeneic marrow grafting using HL-A matched donor-recipient sibling pairs. *Trans. Assoc. Am. Phys.*, in press.

Thompson, M. W., McCulloch, E. A., Siminovitch, L., and Till, J. E., 1966. The cellular basis for the defect in haemopoiesis in flexed-tail mice. I. Nature and persistence of the defect. *Brit. J. Haematol.* 12:152.

Trentin, J. J., 1956. Effect of X-ray dose on mortality and skin transplantability in mice receiving F₁ hybrid marrow. *Proc. Soc. Exptl. Biol. Med.* 93:98.

Trentin, J. J., 1957. Whole-body X-ray and bone marrow therapy of leukemia in mice. *Proc. Am. Assoc. Cancer Res.* 2:256.

Uphoff, D. E., 1963. Genetic factors influencing irradiation protection by bone marrow. III. Midlethal irradiation of inbred mice. *J. Natl. Cancer Inst.* 30:1115.

van Bekkum, D. W., and deVries, M. J., 1967. *Radiation Chimeras*, Logos Press, London, pp. 1-277.

van Bekkum, D. W., and Vos, O., 1957. Immunological aspects of homo- and heterologous bone marrow transplantation in irradiated animals. *J. Cell. Comp. Physiol.* 50:139.

Van Putten, L. M., 1964. Thymectomy: Effect on secondary disease in radiation chimeras. *Science* 145:935.

Van Putten, L. M., van Bekkum, D. W., deVries, M. J., and Balner, H., 1967. The effect of preceding blood transfusions on the fate of homologous bone marrow grafts in lethally irradiated monkeys. *Blood* 30:749.

Winner, H. L., and Hurley, R., 1964. *Candida albicans*, Little, London, pp. 1-306.

Wintrobe, M. M., 1967. *Clinical Hematology*, 6th ed., Lea and Febiger, Philadelphia, pp. 795-796.

Wiskott, A., 1937. Familiärer, angeborener, morbus warlhoffi? *Mschr. Kinderheilk.* 68:212.

Yankee, R. A., Grumet, F. C., and Rogentine, G. N., 1969. Platelet transfusion therapy: The selection of compatible platelet donors for refractory patients by lymphocyte HL-A typing. *New Engl. J. Med.* 281:1208.

Voisin, G. A., Kinsky, R., and Maillard, J., 1968. Protection against homologous disease in hybrid mice by passive and active immunological enhancement facilitation. *Transplantation* 6:187.

Index